INSTITUTE FOR HEALTH INFORMATICS AND FACULTY OF LAW
UNIVERSITY OF WALES, ABERYSTWYTH

HOW TO KEEP A
CLINICAL
CONFIDENCE

A Summary of Law & Guidance on
Maintaining the Patient's Privacy

LONDON: HMSO

ISBN 0 11 701832 5

Authors:
Bryden Darley BSc
Antony Griew MB BS, MSc(Soc Med), MFCM(Irel)
Kathryn McLoughlin BA
John Williams, LLB (Wales), LLB (Cantab), Barrister-at-Law

Institute for Health Informatics and Faculty of Law,
University of Wales, Aberystwyth

Abstract:
This book is concerned with the security issues related to health
care. The work summarises the legal, ethical, and regulatory
position in England and Wales regarding the collection and use of
sensitive information by the health care professions. Appendices
cover social care and forthcoming European Community legislation.

The authors would like to thank Rosemary Currell, Dr Peter Edwards, Gerry Gold, and the other members of the Institute for Health Informatics, as well as Dr David Bellamy and Mr Peter Smith at the Department of Health's Policy Division, for their support and constructive comments. Particular indebtedness is due to Rosemary, and to Jane Durbin, who assisted the authors with many hours of proof reading.

In relation to section 4 (Guidelines) the following organisations were consulted concerning the accuracy of the sections relating to the guidance they have issued, which we have quoted herein. We are grateful to them for their comments, and particularly to those who were kind enough to take the time to comment more generally on the documentation they were sent. Those changes which they recommended, and which we found appropriate (the great majority), have been incorporated into the text, but any errors which remain are of course the sole responsibility of the authors.

> The General Medical Council
> The Medical Defence Union
> The Medical Protection Society
> The United Kingdom Central Council for Nursing, Midwifery and Health Visiting
> The Royal College of Obstetricians and Gynaecologists
> The Health Visitors Association
> The British Paediatric Association
> The British Psychological Society
> The Royal College of Nursing
> The Council for the Professions Supplementary to Medicine
> The British Medical Association
> Mr J D Williams (a personal view of the guidelines from the viewpoint of social work)

The work leading to the production of this book arose from the requirements of a project funded by the Welsh Office.

Please note that where one gender is used, it should be taken to include the other, wherever this is appropriate. "He or she" tends to interrupt the flow of the sentence, and has therefore been truncated.

CONTENTS

Commissions to develop standards for handling clinical data and the information derived from them, form a substantial proportion of the work of the Institute for Health Informatics at the University of Wales in Aberystwyth. Attention to confidentiality and the authorisation of access to such data is clearly an important issue to be addressed, and grows daily in public and political awareness. The Institute therefore decided, as part of one of its commissions, to attempt to develop a general strategy towards the protection of sensitive data. The first attempt to gain a degree of public and professional consensus regarding the rules to be applied within such a strategy, has recently been sent to the bodies controlling the activities of the various health professions for their initial observations, and to open the debate.

To be able to produce this strategy it was clearly necessary to seek factual source material. Failure to conform to requirements, both of the law and of the guidance issued by the professions involved in health care, would doom it to instant oblivion. This was the genesis of the present work. The authors could find no single source from which to obtain this information. As our efforts neared completion, it became clear that what we were creating was not simply a means to our primary goal. Others saw our compilation as a reference source of value to their own concerns. We were repeatedly requested for copies, however incomplete and unvalidated. It was apparent that our needs were likely to be repeated throughout the health care world, and possibly beyond.

This book is intended to give the reader seeking to implement an activity requiring the control of confidential material an overview of the field, and guidance to areas where more detailed study would be productive in the specific circumstances obtaining.

Readers should note that this book has been written to be as readable as is consonant with accuracy. Section 3, on Statute Law, cannot therefore be taken to be legally definitive, since virtually all of the terminology used in the drafting of the legislation described has been reworded to make it clear, rather than watertight.

Two areas outside of health care are of clear importance to those practising within it. The first is social care. The interaction between doctors, nurses and social workers is close, if at times uneasy. It is important to acknowledge this, and to take account of the guidance given by the social work professions regarding confidentiality. The second is the fact that a proposed Directive from the European Commission is in its second draft, and its passage, if unchanged in substance, would materially affect English law. We have therefore provided appendices on each of these issues.

The bibliography which ends this work is not intended to be comprehensive. It should nonetheless give adequate guidance to those wishing to delve deeper into this important area of social and legislative activity.

Bryden Darley, Antony Griew, Kathryn McLoughlin, John Williams

2.1 A Dictionary Definition

The terms *"confidential"* and *"confidentiality"* are defined in the Oxford English Dictionary (compact edn., Book Club Associates 1979) as:

Confidential a. [f. L. *confidentia* CONFIDENCE + AL. Cf. F. *confidentiel*.]

1. Confident, bold (obs., rare).

2. Of the nature of confidence; spoken or written in confidence; characterised by the communication of secrets or private matters.

   Confidential communication, a communication made between parties who stand in a confidential relation to each other, and therefore privileged in law. *Confidential relation*, the relation existing between a lawyer and his client, between guardian and ward.

   e.g. 1883 *Manch. Guard.* 12 Oct. 5/6 The report . . . was to be made . . . without any confidential mention of the names of persons.

3. Betokening private intimacy, or the confiding of private secrets.

   e.g. 1884 F. M. CRAWFORD *Rom. Singer* I. 29 Nino became very confidential.

4. Enjoying the confidence of another person; entrusted with secrets; charged with secret service.

   e.g. 1856 FROUDE *Hist. Eng.* (1858) I.ii. 133 Confidential persons were despatched into Italy to obtain an interview . . . with the pope.

Confidentiality [f. prec. + ITY]

Confidential quality; state of being confidential.

e.g. 1834 W. TAYLOR in Robberds *Mem.* II. 566 The employment of an amanuensis would abolish all real confidentiality in our correspondence. 1881 W.C. RUSSELL *Ocean Free Lance* II. 110 [Her] soft eyes and winning confidentiality of manner.

2.2 The General Rule

The General Medical Council's (GMC 1993) *"Professional conduct and discipline: fitness to practice"* states that subject to certain conditions, *"Patients are entitled to expect that the information about themselves or others which a doctor learns during the course of a medical consultation, investigation or treatment, will remain confidential. Doctors therefore have a duty not to disclose to any third party information about an individual that they have learned in their professional capacity, directly from a patient or indirectly"*. Confidentiality is the privilege of the patient, and not the health care professional. Consequently, it is the patient who has the right to waive that privilege and consent to the disclosure of information.

2.3 Confidentiality - The Common Law

The duty of confidentiality is one that has been developed by the judiciary in a series of cases dealing with a wide range of confidential relationships. Although the duty of confidence may arise by virtue of a contractual relationship, the common law has recognised the importance of providing protection for confidential relationships in the absence of such a specific relationship. The law was re-affirmed by the House of Lords in *Attorney General* v *Guardian Newspapers Ltd (No2)*[1], the so called *Spycatcher Case*. In his judgment Lord Goff accepted the "broad principle" that a duty of confidence arises in the following circumstances:

(a)   information is confidential

(b)   it comes to the knowledge of a person (the confidant) in circumstances where he or she has notice, or is held to have agreed, that the information is confidential, with the effect that it would be just that he or she should be precluded from disclosing the information

(c)   it is in the public interest that the confidentiality should be protected.

---

[1][1988] 3 All ER 545

There can be little doubt that the doctor/patient relationship is prima facie a confidential one. In *Hunter* v *Mann*[2] Boreham J stated that,

> ". . . *the doctor is under a duty not to disclose, without the consent of the patient, information which he, the doctor, has gained in his professional capacity.*"

Confidentiality is an implied component of the doctor/patient relationship. Patients have a legitimate expectation, protected by the common law, that the information they give to their doctors will be kept confidential and will not enter the public domain. Thus the first two requirements of the test propounded by Lord Goff are easily satisfied in the doctor/patient relationship. It should be noted that this duty of confidentiality is not an absolute one. Statute as well as the common law recognises exceptions.

The more difficult issue is the third requirement laid down by Lord Goff. It must be in the public interest that confidentiality is protected. Judges have had great difficulty in defining the public interest. One particular dilemma that often arises is where there are two competing public interests; which one is to prevail?

To argue that there is one "public interest" is misleading. For example, in *D* v *NSPCC*[3] there was a public interest in encouraging people to report cases of suspected child abuse which supported the need for confidentiality; there was also a competing interest, namely the need to have proper regard for the administration of justice.

The public interest justification for the confidentiality of the doctor/patient relationship was stated by Rose J in *X* v *Y*[4] as follows,

> "*In the long run, preservation of confidentiality is the only way of securing public health; otherwise doctors will be discredited*

---

[2][1974] 2 All ER 414   [3][1977] 1 All ER 589   [4][1988] 2 All ER 648

as a source of education, for future individual patients will not come forward if doctors are going to squeal on them. Consequently, confidentiality is vital to secure public as well as private health, for unless those infected come forward they cannot be counselled and self-treatment does not provide the best care . . . "

X v *Y* is one of a series of cases in which the public interest dimension was explored by the courts. A newspaper had received information, in breach of confidence, that two general practitioners diagnosed as HIV positive were continuing to practice. The Health Authority sought an injunction preventing the newspaper from revealing the identity of the doctors. It was argued by the newspaper that it was in the public interest that patients were aware that their doctor was HIV positive. However, this argument was rejected by Rose J who held that the negligible risk to the patients could not outweigh the important public interest in people seeking medical help if they thought that there was a chance that they were HIV positive.

A different conclusion was reached by the Court of Appeal in *W* v *Egdell*[5]. The question before the court was whether a report prepared by a consultant psychiatrist for a patient detained under the Mental Health Act 1983 could be disclosed to a third party. The patient was detained in a secure hospital without limit; he had killed five people. Originally the report was prepared at the behest of the patient's solicitor who was preparing an application to a Mental Health Review Tribunal. The application was withdrawn largely because the consultant's report was unfavourable. However, the consultant disclosed the report to the hospital which sent a copy to the Secretary of State. The Court found that the balance of public interest lay in the *restricted* disclosure of the report to the hospital and to the Secretary of State as they had responsibility for public safety. It is essential to note that the Court only sanctioned a restricted disclosure of the report.

[5][1990] 1 All ER 835

These two cases illustrate the courts' approach to the issue of public interest. Both cases emphasise the importance of the public interest in confidentiality and consider exceptions as a rarity. In *Egdell* the Court referred to the General Medical Council's *Blue Book* (1993). Although the rules in the *Blue Book* do not have the force of law, they are extremely useful to courts in determining acceptable professional conduct. Rule 81(g) deals with the public interest defence. It states,

> "*Rarely, disclosure may be justified on the ground that it is in the public interest which, in certain circumstances . . . might override the doctor's duty to maintain the patient's confidence.*"

The *Blue Book* cites as an example a police investigation of a grave or serious crime. Rule 82 required a doctor who discloses confidential information to justify the action.

The common law provides considerable protection for the public interest in the maintenance of the confidentiality of the doctor/patient relationship. Only where there is an overriding public interest contrary to the one stated by Rose J in *X* v *Y* will the courts contemplate sanctioning a breach of that relationship.

The common law will also sanction breaches of confidentiality where they accord with good medical practice. The use of the *Blue Book* in the *Egdell* case suggests that disclosures falling within rule 81 would be respected by law. Nevertheless, caution must be exercised when considering disclosure, as regard must be had to that predominant public interest, which the common law recognises as central to the relationship. The Blue Book states that if in doubt doctors should consult their medical defence association.

If confidential information is disclosed contrary to the common law rules discussed above and without statutory justification, the aggrieved patient will have recourse to law. Such action is in addition to any disciplinary action that may be taken against the doctor concerned. If a patient wishes to take the matter to law he or she may bring an action for breach of confidence. As Brazier points out, an action for breach of confidence has much more relevance in a commercial setting where loss as a result of breach is more easily quantified in money terms.[6] For the patient whose confidential medical records have been disclosed unlawfully financial loss may well be nominal whereas injury to pride, status and reputation may be considerable. Damage to these less quantifiable injuries may give rise to only nominal damages being awarded by the court, although each case will have to be decided on its own facts. Clearly where the patient suffered direct financial loss (for example job loss) this will be more easily compensated by the courts.

Damages may be difficult and costly to obtain, and may be nominal. However, the action can be used as a means of *preventing* a future disclosure in breach of confidence. If the patient suspects or knows that a doctor is intending to disclose without authority, an action may be brought to prevent that disclosure. At the hearing the court will, of course, consider whether the proposed disclosure falls within either the common law or statutory exceptions.

---

[6]*Medicine, Patient and the Law*, Margaret Brazier, Penguin, 1992.

3.0 STATUTORY REQUIREMENTS AND CONSTRAINTS

This section contains summaries of legislation that affects the security, access, confidentiality, disclosure, and transfer of medical information. Three Acts that came into existence specifically to make provisions in this area, the Data Protection Act 1984, the Access to Medical Reports Act 1988, and the Access to Health Records Act 1990 are explained first. They are followed by such other legislation as impacts upon the way in which medical information can be used.

3.1 Data Protection Act 1984

The Data Protection Act 1984 was intended *"to regulate the use of automatically processed information relating to individuals and the provision of services in respect of such information"*. There are eight data protection principles, which are listed below, seven applying to the data user, and the last to computer bureaux.

3.1.1 The Principles

1. The information to be contained in personal data shall be obtained, and personal data shall be processed, fairly and lawfully.

2. Personal data shall be held only for one or more specified and lawful purposes.

3. Personal data held for any purpose or purposes shall not be used or disclosed in any manner incompatible with that purpose or those purposes.

4. Personal data held for any purpose or purposes shall be adequate, relevant and not excessive in relation to that purpose or those purposes.

5. Personal data shall be accurate and, where necessary, kept up to date.

6. Personal data held for any purpose or purposes shall not be kept for longer than is necessary for that purpose or those purposes.

7.   An individual shall be entitled -

        (a) at reasonable intervals and without undue delay or expense -

             (i) to be informed by any data user whether he holds personal data of which that individual is the subject and

             (ii) to access any such data held by a data user; and

        (b) where appropriate, to have such data corrected or erased.

8.   Appropriate security measures shall be taken against unauthorised access to, or alteration, disclosure or destruction of, personal data and against accidental loss or destruction of personal data.

It is worth noting that the provisions of the Act do not apply to the records of deceased persons, and that this conflicts with the draft E.C. legislation outlined in Appendix C, and with much professional guidance (see section 4).

3.1.2 Exemptions

The Secretary of State may make an order under section 29 of the Act (Part IV Exemptions - Health and Social Work), stating that the data user need not give access to the data subject if in the opinion of the user the information would seriously harm the physical or mental health of the individual concerned, or if the information would identify another person who has not consented to the disclosure of his or her identity (unless the individual is a practitioner and has supplied the information in question in that capacity). The judgement in such cases rests with the data user, who should be advised by a health professional.

In guidance offered by the Department of Health it is made clear that information should be withheld only in exceptional circumstances.

3.1.3 The Subject Access Modification (Health) Order 1987

This order was made under section 29 of the Act, and gives a doctor the right to withhold data from a patient if he feels that it would cause serious harm to the patient's physical or mental health. However, no definition is given as to what constitutes serious harm.

3.2 Access To Medical Reports Act 1988

This act was specifically introduced *"to establish a right of access by individuals to reports relating to themselves provided by medical practitioners for employment or insurance purposes and to make provision for related matters"*. The Act can broadly be considered in four parts, namely: right of access; consent to the supplying of the report; correction of errors; exemptions.

3.2.1 Right of Access

An individual has the right to access any medical report relating to him or herself which is to be, or has been, supplied by the medical practitioner for employment or insurance purposes. The individual if he wishes to exercise this right must, before the report is supplied to a third party, tell the practitioner of his intent.

Only the exemptions specified in the Act can deny the patient access to all or part of a report.

3.2.2 Consent to the Supplying of the Report

The patient always has the right to stop the practitioner from supplying the report to a third party. If the patient does not ask to see the report before it is sent, or if the patient asks to see the report before it is supplied, and then 21 days elapse since the request for access was made without the individual contacting the practitioner, he has in these circumstances given implicit consent for the supply of the report to a third party.

However, if the patient does view the report, either in its entirety or not (according to the exemptions part of the Act) within the 21-day time limit, he may stop the supply of that report to a third party.

3.2.3 Correction of Errors

The individual is entitled, before giving consent to the supply of the report, to request the medical practitioner to amend any part of the report which the individual considers to be incorrect or misleading. In this eventuality two courses of action are open to the practitioner, namely:

(a)   to accede to the request, and amend the report accordingly,

        or

(b)   to refuse to amend the report, in which case a statement of the individual's views in respect to the report shall be attached to the report.

3.2.4 Exemptions

If any information contained within the report would, in the opinion of the medical practitioner, be likely to cause serious harm to the physical or mental health of the individual, or others, or would indicate the intentions of the practitioner in respect of the individual, the practitioner is within his rights not to give the individual access to parts or all of the report in question. In addition, any part of the report that would be likely to reveal information about another person who has supplied information to the practitioner about the individual, cannot be disclosed to the individual unless:

(a)   the person supplying the information has consented,

        or

(b)   the person supplying the information is a health professional and the information was supplied in that capacity.

3.3 Access To Health Records Act 1990

This Act was introduced in 1990 and is essentially the same as the Data Protection Act, but extends the subject access provisions to include manually compiled records. The Act came into force on the 1st November 1991 and only relates to records created on or after this date.

3.3.1 Access

An application for access to an individual's health records can be made by a number of different people, namely:

(a)   the patient

(b)   a person authorised in writing to make the application on the patient's behalf

(c)   the guardian of a minor

(d)   a person appointed by the court to manage the affairs of a patient deemed incapable

(e)   where the patient has died, the patient's personal representative and any person who may have a claim arising out of the patient's death.

3.3.2 Exemptions to the Right of Access

Access to part or all of the record may be refused in certain circumstances. If the applicant is a minor, the holder must be satisfied that he or she is capable of understanding the nature of the application before any disclosure is made. In addition, if a parent, person with parental responsibility or, in Scotland, a guardian, applies for access to the minor's record, the holder can only comply if the minor has given consent, or if in the holder's opinion, access would be in the best interests of the patient and the patient is considered incapable of understanding the nature of the application.

If the patient has died the personal representatives or claimants do not have an automatic right of access to the deceased's record. If the record in question includes a note made at the patient's request that he did not wish access to be given on such an application, then disclosure cannot be made by the holder. Also, if the holder is of the opinion that information relating to the deceased is not relevant to any claim being made, then he need not disclose that information.

Other exemptions to the patient's right of access are similar to those in the Data Protection Act and the Access to Health Records Act. The only addition is that if information is provided by the patient in the expectation that it will not be disclosed, or information is obtained as a result of an examination or investigation to which the patient consents, in the expectation that it will not be disclosed, then no other applicant can be allowed access to those parts of the record.

3.3.3 The Correction of Inaccurate Health Records

The provisions under this Act for the correction of incorrect, misleading or incomplete records are again similar to the Data Protection Act and the Access to Medical Reports Act. If the applicant feels that information contained in the record is inaccurate and requests that the record be amended accordingly, the holder may make the necessary correction. If in the holder's opinion the request is not valid, then the record will not be amended, but a note will be attached to the record detailing the applicant's view. In both cases a copy of the correction or note must be supplied to the applicant.

3.4 Abortion Act 1967

A registered medical practitioner carrying out an abortion must under the Abortion Act 1967 give notice of the termination, along with other information relating to it. The information must be passed in England to the Department of Health, in Wales to the Welsh Office, and in Scotland the Scottish Office (the Act does not extend to Northern Ireland) within seven days of the termination, on the form specified in the Act. The patient has no right to restrict the disclosure to those authorities of information relating to the termination. The notice is sent specifically to the Chief Medical Officer for each country.

3.5 Access To Personal Files Act 1987

See Appendix B Section 3.

3.6 Children Act 1989

The Children Act 1989 stipulates that the guardian ad litem of a child has the right *"at all reasonable times to examine and take copies of"* any of the records relating to the child in question made under the Act or the Local Social Services Act 1970, and held by a local authority's Social Services department. In addition, the guardian ad litem may use a copy of the record to make a report to a court, or to use as evidence in any court proceedings. (For fuller treatment of this issue, see Appendix B).

3.7 Computer Misuse Act 1990

This Act came into force to make provision for securing computer programs and data against unauthorised access or modification. Authorised users have permission to access certain applications and data. If those users go beyond specified bounds then an offence has been committed. The Act makes provision for accidental transgressions, as well as covering fraud, extortion, and blackmail.

3.8 Public Health (Control of Diseases) Act 1984

Sections 10 and 11 of this Act relate to notifiable disease and food poisoning. The Act requires a qualified medical practitioner to send a certificate to the Medical Officer of Health of the district stating:

(a)   the name, age and sex of the patient and the address of the premises where the patient is presently staying

(b)   the disease, or particulars of the food poisoning, and the date of its onset

(c)   if the premises is a hospital, then: the day on which the patient was admitted; the address from which the patient came; and, in the opinion of the person giving the certificate, the disease or poisoning suspected.

It is then the responsibility of the Officer who receives the certificate to send a copy within forty-eight hours to:

(a)   the Health Authority whose area covers the afflicted premises, and

(b)   if the patient is hospitalised and came from premises outside the area of the Local Authority, to the proper officer for the district from which the patient was sent, to the Health Authority concerned, and if appropriate to the officer of the relevant Port Health Authority.

Certificates can also be issued by practitioners practising in the affected area if they believe that one or a group of people, though not suffering from the disease, is carrying an organism that is capable of causing it, and that it is in the public interest that those persons should be medically examined.

The notifiable diseases in England and Wales, Scotland, and Northern Ireland are listed below.

3.8.1 Notifiable Diseases in England and Wales

Acute encephalitis	Leprosy	Scarlet fever
Acute meningitis	Leptospirosis	Smallpox
Acute poliomyelitis	Malaria	Tetanus
Amoebic dysentery	Marburgh virus disease	Tuberculosis
Anthrax	Measles	Typhoid fever
Cholera	Meningitis meningococcal	Typhus
Diphtheria	Ophthalmia neonatorum	Viral haemorrhagic fever
Dysentery	Paratyphoid fever	Viral hepatitis
Erysipelas	Plague	Whooping cough
Fever	Rabies	Yellow fever
Food poisoning	Relapsing fever	Rubella

3.8.2 Notifiable Diseases in Northern Ireland

All of the above.

| Additions: | Chicken pox | Legionnaire's disease |
| | Hepatitis B | Gastro-enteritis (under two years) |

3.8.3 Notifiable Diseases in Scotland

All of the above except Amoebic dysentery.

Additions:	Legionellosis	Puerperal fever
	Lyme disease	Toxoplasmosis [11]
	Membranous croup	

3.9 Human Fertilisation And Embryology Act 1990

The Act applies to the Human Fertilisation and Embryology Authority, which is required to keep a register which contains information with regard to human fertilisation and embryology if it falls within three areas:

(a) the provision of treatment services for identifiable individuals, or

(b) the keeping or use of the gametes of any identifiable individual or of an embryo taken from any identifiable woman, or

(c) it shows that an identifiable individual was born in consequence of the treatment.

3.9.1 Disclosure of Information

A person eighteen or over has the right by notice to the Authority to require it to comply with a request for disclosure of information if:

(a) the information contained in the register shows that the applicant was, or may have been, born in consequence of treatment, and

(b) the applicant has been given suitable opportunity to receive proper counselling about the implications of compliance with the request.

In addition the applicant can ask the Authority whether or not the information contained in the register shows that someone other than his known parent might be his genetic parent. The regulations do state, however, that the identity of the person whose gametes have been used, or from whom an embryo has been taken, do not have to be identified if donation occurred before the Act was implemented.

The applicant may also seek information concerning his or her intended spouse to check whether they are related.

3.9.2 Restrictions on the Disclosure of Information

No employee of the Authority is permitted to disclose any of the following information:

(a)   any information contained in the register, and

(b)   any other information obtained on terms or in circumstances requiring it to be held in confidence.

Point (a) above does not apply to a disclosure of information if it is made:

- to a person who is another employee of the Authority, or
- to a person to whom a licence applies for the purposes of his functions, or
- where no individual to whom the information relates can be identified, or
- to the Registrar General.

Point (b), above does not apply if it is:

- made to a person who is an employee of the Authority,
- made with the consent of the person or persons whose confidence would otherwise be protected, or
- lawfully available to the public before the disclosure is made.

3.9.3 Disclosure in the Interests of Justice

Before a court the question as to whether a person is or is not the parent of a child can be determined by the disclosure of fertilisation and embryological information. The court must decide before making the disclosure whether or not the interests of justice require it. It must take into account any representations made by an individual who may be affected by the disclosure, and the welfare of the child, if under 18 years old, and the welfare of any other person under that age who might be affected by the disclosure.

3.10 Human Organ Transplant Act 1989

Under this Act, the Secretary of State may make regulations requiring specified persons to supply to a specified authority information about transplants that have been, or are proposed to be, carried out in Great Britain, using organs removed from living or dead persons. The authority is required to keep a register of the information supplied. Any person failing to comply with these regulations is guilty of an offence and is liable to prosecution.

3.11 Mental Health Act 1983

Under sections 13 and 14 of the Act it is the duty of a local Social Services department, if required by the nearest relative of a patient, to direct an approved social worker to consider the patient's case with a view to making an application for the patient's admission to hospital. If, in the opinion of the social worker, a referral to hospital is not appropriate then the nearest relative must be informed in writing of the decision and the reasons behind it.

If the patient is to be admitted to hospital, it is then the responsibility of the management of the hospital to notify the Social Services department for the area in which the patient resided immediately before admission, so that the department can send a social worker to interview the patient and provide a report on his or her social circumstances.

3.12 Misuse of Drugs Act 1971

Section 17 of the Act relates to actions that can be carried out in an area if there seems to be a problem in connection with the misuse of dangerous or otherwise harmful drugs.

3.12.1 The Notice

If a social problem is seen to exist it is within the powers of the
Home Secretary to issue a written notice to any doctor, pharmacist,
or retail pharmacy business (within the meaning of the Medicines
Act 1968) in or near the area, requiring particulars of the quanti-
ties in which, and the number and frequency of the occasions on
which, harmful drugs were:

(a)   (in the case of a doctor) prescribed, administered or
        supplied by him, or

(b)   (in the case of a pharmacist) supplied by him, or

(c)   (in the case of a person carrying on a retail pharmacy
        business) supplied in the course of business at any
        premises specified in the notice.

If a notice under this section is served on a person carrying on a
retail pharmacy business, it may require him to furnish the names
and addresses of doctors whose prescriptions for the specified
dangerous drugs he dispensed. It shall not require any person
to reveal the identity of any person for whom the drug has been
prescribed or supplied.

3.13 NHS Act 1977

The requirements of section 124 of the NHS Act 1977 relate to the
notification of births and deaths. For births and deaths it is the
responsibility of the Registrar to give the required information to
the prescribed medical officer of the District Health Authority. This
information relates to the particulars of each birth or death which
occurred in the Authority's district, as entered in the register of
births and deaths.

Section 124 also requires the giving of **notice** of a birth to the
prescribed medical officer of the DHA in which the birth takes
place. In the case of every child born, it is the duty of the child's
father (if at the time of birth he resides in the premises where the
child is born), and of any person in attendance upon the mother at

the time of, or within six hours of, the birth to **notify** the pre-scribed medical officer of the birth. The Registrar will have access at all reasonable times to this information.

The Act does not affect the duty to **register** births and deaths under the Births and Deaths Registration Act 1953. This Act covers both live births and stillbirths as defined in the Stillbirths (Definition) Act 1992. Certain persons are identified as "qualified persons" and are under a duty to inform the Registrar, and to sign the register. Normally this duty falls upon a relative or member of the household. However, a doctor or other healthcare professional present at the birth or death, will also be a "qualified person" and may therefore be under a duty to provide information to the Registrar.

There is no statutory requirement for a doctor to report deaths, but he or she is advised to inform the coroner in the following circum-stances:

- Sudden or unexpected deaths:
    - (a) the doctor cannot certify the real (as opposed to the immediate) cause of death, or
    - (b) where the doctor has not attended in the last illness.
- Abortions - other than spontaneous.
- Accidents and injuries which contributed to the cause of death.
- Anaesthetics and operations - deaths while under anaesthetic and deaths following an operation.
- Crime or suspected crime.
- Drugs, therapeutic mishap, and addiction and abuse.
- Ill treatment, starvation and neglect
- Industrial disease deaths arising out of a patient's employment.
- Infant deaths if in any way questionable.
- Patients detained under the Mental Health Act 1983.
- Pensioners receiving a disability pension when the death may be connected with the pensionable disability.

- Persons in legal custody (prisons, remand centres, approved schools etc.)
- Poisoning - all causes.
- Septicaemias which have originated from an injury.
- Stillbirths where:
  - (a) there is any possibility of the child having been born alive, or
  - (b) where there may be cause for suspicion.

3.14 Venereal Diseases Act 1917

These regulations require every Health Authority to take adequate steps to ensure that information capable of identifying an individual, obtained by health authority officers with respect to persons examined or treated for any sexually transmitted disease, shall not be disclosed, except to another doctor or to someone who is employed under his direction, in connection with the treatment or the prevention of the spread of such diseases. Information shall not be disclosed except for these purposes.

3.15 Police And Criminal Evidence Act 1984

Section 9 states that a police officer may apply to a circuit judge for an order to access documentation classified under the Act as "excluded material" (which could, e.g., include medical records), providing that notice of the application is given and that the judge is satisfied that various conditions can all be met. These are that:

- (a) There must be reasonable grounds for believing that there is material on the premises that is specified in the application
- (b) There must be some statutory authority enacted prior to the Police and Criminal Evidence Act (and not invalidated by this act), which would have authorised such a search
- (c) The issue of a warrant under the Act is appropriate.

Section 13 provides powers for the general seizure of documents to a police officer who is already on the premises and it is theoretically possible for medical records to be seized in this way.

3.16 Prevention Of Terrorism (Temporary Provisions) Act 1984

The Prevention of Terrorism Act defines terrorism as "... *the use of violence for political ends and includes any use of violence for the purpose of putting the public or any section of the public in fear*". A person can be guilty of a criminal offence "*if he has information which he knows or believes might be of material assistance*", and if he fails "*without reasonable excuse*" to disclose this information to the appropriate authority.

The Act empowers the Police to obtain any documentation held by any individual or organisation that could be used as evidence against the accused. This right of access can be exercised with or without a search warrant.

3.16.1 Powers of Search With a Warrant

A warrant authorises the applicant (and any other members of the police force) entry to premises, if necessary by force, and to search the premises and every person in it. Anything found that an officer has reasonable grounds to suspect can be used as evidence can be seized.

3.16.2 Powers of Search Without a Warrant

An officer may under the Act arrest or stop any person for the purposes of searching the individual for articles or documents which may constitute evidence.

3.17 Road Traffic Act 1972

During court proceedings for a motoring offence, if it appears that the defendant may be suffering from any disease or physical disability which might effect his or her driving ability, and therefore would be a danger to the public, the court must notify the

Secretary of State. The information to be contained in a notification will be determined by the Secretary of State.

3.18 Supreme Court Act 1981

The Supreme Court Act 1981 was introduced to deal with disclosures of records for the purpose of litigation in England and Wales. Section 34 of the Act states that it *"applies to any proceedings in the High Court in which a claim is made in respect of personal injuries to a person, or in respect of a person's death"*.

3.18.1 The Order

Under the Act it is within the power of the court to order a person who is not party to the proceedings but who it appears to the court may possess documents relevant to the claim to:

(a) disclose to the court whether he actually does have the documents in his possession, and

(b) produce the documents to the applicant or (according to the conditions of the order), to:

(i) the applicant's legal advisor, or

(ii) to the applicant's legal advisers and any medical or other professional adviser of the applicant, or

(iii) if the applicant has no legal adviser, to any medical or other professional adviser of the applicant.

3.18.2 The Provisions of the Order

The order may be made in respect of one or more of the following:

(a) inspection, photocopying, preservation, custody and detention of property (which need not be the property of any party involved in the proceedings), which is the subject-matter of any question arising in the proceedings

(b) the taking of samples of any property mentioned above, and the carrying out of any experiment on, or with, such property.

The High Court will only make an order if it would not be likely to be injurious to the public interest.

4.1 The Health Care Professional's Duty Of Confidentiality

The Medical Defence Union (MDU) uses the following definition for the word confidential:

> "*spoken or written in confidence; entrusted with secrets; charged with secret tasks*". (in O'Donovan 1992)

The need for confidentiality was recognised as far back as the 5th century BC. The Hippocratic oath states:

> "*whatever, in connection with my professional practice or not in connection with it, I see or hear in the life of men, which ought not to be spoken abroad, I will not divulge as reckoning that all such should be kept secret.*" (in O'Donovan 1992)

This was restated in 1947 in the declaration of Geneva:

> "*I will respect the secrets which are confided in me, even after the patient has died.*" (in O'Donovan 1992)

The freedom of speech between a patient and doctor is central to, and an essential part of, the diagnosis of a patient. Indeed, some would add that the doctor's surgery can be likened to the confessional. The United Kingdom Central Council (UKCC 1987), the governing body for nurses, midwives, and health visitors, states that the focal word in its definition of confidentiality is the word "*trust*", and puts forward the view that ". . . *without this trust, no therapeutic relationship can be developed or maintained between the health care worker and the patient or client*". The Medical Protection Society (MPS 1992) adds that in English law there is no general statutory duty of confidentiality. However, most Lawyers would agree that the term confidentiality is ". . . *an implied term of the contract between the doctor and his patient*", and that ". . . *unauthorised disclosure of professional secrets would be a breach of contract giving grounds for civil proceedings*" (UKCC 1987).

That duty is enforceable by injunction, by a civil claim for damages, or by rules formulated by bodies with statutory powers to regulate the profession (e.g. the GMC) from whom, it may be argued, medical practitioners have more to fear.[7] The UKCC (1987) states: "*. . . confidentiality is a rule with certain exceptions. There is no statutory right of confidentiality; but there is also no bar to an aggrieved individual bringing a common law case before a civil court alleging breach of confidentiality and seeking financial recompense*". It should be noted that while there is no general statutory right, there are some limited statutory provisions (for example, in the Venereal Diseases Regulations 1917 and in the Human Fertilisation and Embryology Act, 1990–q.v.). In the NHS, a Health Authority employee is accountable to the patient, to the law, and to the employer, and, whether he is a clinician or not, litigation is of concern. The British Medical Association guidelines (BMA 1992) confirm that: "*At present there is no statutory right to sue another person for breach of confidentiality, and the legal position can only be defined from a study of decided court cases and academic comment*". A patient would have to prove:

(a)   that there was a duty of confidentiality, and

(b)   that the duty of confidentiality was breached.

Case law has shown that courts will generally enforce a duty of confidentiality where:

(a)   information is not a matter of public knowledge, or

(b)   information is given to an individual in a situation where there is an obligation not to disclose the information without consent, or

(c)   where protecting confidentiality is in the public interest.

4.2 Information To Colleagues

The GMC believes that information may be shared with other registered medical professionals who assist with the patient's clinical management. The extent to which information may be

---

[7]Letter from the MPS 28 February 1994

shared with other health care professionals concerned with the patient's health (e.g. dentists, nurses and the other professions associated with medicine) is decided upon by the clinician. It is the clinician's duty to ensure that those with whom information is shared appreciate the rule of professional secrecy, although it would probably be fair to say that those health care professionals receiving the information will usually work according to their own profession's established code of ethics.

Where it is necessary to share information between members of a health care team, it is again up to the individual clinician to make a decision as to what information he is willing to disclose to other members of the team.

4.3 Disclosure Of Information After Death

The extent to which information can be disclosed after a person's death depends upon the circumstances, but it is the consensus, amongst health care professionals and professional and statutory bodies such as the GMC, that a patient's death does not release a doctor from his obligation to maintain confidentiality. Criteria for decisions on when information might be disclosed after death include:

(a)   the period of time which has elapsed,

(b)   the nature of the information disclosed,

(c)   the extent to which it has already appeared in published material,

(d)   statutory rights of access under the Access to Health Records Act, 1990.

Where the information is sought by a third party about the deceased patient, the consent of all personal representatives should be sought (i.e. his executors and those who take out letters of administration). The MDU (O'Donovan 1992) would add that when a patient dies intestate, the next of kin should be consulted.

4.4 An Ill Or Mentally Incapable Person

A doctor may deem that a patient is incapable of giving or withholding consent for disclosure, for reasons of immaturity, abuse
or neglect, or due to illness or mental incapacity, and cannot fully
appreciate the implications of the advice being sought. In these
circumstances, the GMC (1993) states that *"the patient's interests
are paramount and will usually require the doctor to disclose
relevant information to an appropriate, responsible person or an
officer of a statutory agency"*. As always a practitioner must be
prepared to justify any breach of confidentiality to his professional
peers.

4.5 Epidemiology

Epidemiology is the study of the determinants (aetiology) and
distribution of disease.

In the United Kingdom the Epidemiologist fulfils three main tasks:

(a)   aetiological research,

(b)   the control of hazards to health, and

(c)   the assessment of the population's need for health care
        (which effectively equates to research into the distri-
        bution of disease).

The doctor's position regarding the release of information for
epidemiological research is not clear. In theory, and to take the
situation to an extreme, information is confidential whether the
identity of the patient is known or not; aggregated or not. However,
because of the obvious value of such data in epidemiological
research, and precisely because of the aggregated and anonymised
nature of most of the data needed, patient data is generally shared
with epidemiologists. The guidance the BMA (1992) offers is as
follows:

> *"Epidemiological research through studies of medical records
> can be extremely valuable. Patients are, however, entitled to*

regard their medical records as confidential to the NHS and should in principle be asked if they consent to their own records being released to research workers. However, there will be occasions when a researcher would find it very difficult to obtain such consent from every individual and the LREC will need to be satisfied that the value of such a project outweighs, in the public interest, the principle that individual consent should be obtained. Where a patient has previously indicated that he or she would not want their records released, then this request should be respected. . . . Certain enquiries and surveys, involving only access to patients records, such as national morbidity surveys and the post marketing surveillance of drugs, which are in the public interest, do not need prior approval of an LREC."

4.6 People Under 16 And Contraception

The current legal position with regard to children under the age of sixteen having the right to consent to treatment was established in *Gillick* v *Norfolk and Wisbech Area Health Authority*[8] (see appendix A section 2). This case was specifically to do with contraceptive advice and treatment, and the ruling clearly stated that competent minors were at liberty to determine their own course of treatment.

However, if the minor is considered to be immature, the latest guidance advises that:

". . . disclosure without consent may be justified where the patient does not have sufficient understanding to appreciate what the advice or treatment being sought may involve, cannot be persuaded to involve an appropriate person in the consultation, and where it would, in the doctor's belief, be essential to the best medical interests of the patient." (BMA 1993).

---

[8][1985] 3 All ER 402 HL

It is stressed by both the GMC and the BMA in their respective codes of conduct, that a doctor must always be prepared to justify any disclosure of confidential information whatever the circumstances.

The House of Lords ruling was accompanied by guidance from Lord Fraser of Tullybelton. The criteria which would justify the doctor proceeding without parental consent were as follows:

- that the girl[9] (although under sixteen years of age) will understand the advice
- that he cannot persuade her to inform her parents, or to allow him to inform her parents, that she is seeking contraceptive advice
- that she is very likely to begin or to continue having sexual intercourse with or without contraceptive treatment
- that, unless she receives contraceptive advice or treatment, her physical or mental health, or both, are likely to suffer
- that her best interests require the doctor to give her contraceptive advice and/or treatment without parental consent.

4.7 Examinations For Insurance Companies And Employers

When performing an examination for an employer or insurance company, the doctor must ensure that the patient is fully aware that he, the doctor, has a duty to the employer (or insurance company) as well as to the patient. This additional duty to a third party does not negate the doctor's responsibility towards the patient.

Doctors should only undertake a commissioned medical examination of a patient after he has ensured that the patient has a clear understanding of the purpose of the examination, or consultation, and has given written consent. A doctor should divulge no secrets

---

[9] The case in question involved the right to contraception for an under age girl, and the judgement was conveyed accordingly.

about a patient unless directed to do so in legally acceptable circumstances. This applies to insurance companies, housing departments, and Social Services departments.

4.8 Nursing, Health Visiting And Midwifery

In *"Managing Nursing Work"*, Vaughan and Pillmore (1989) state that it is often the nurse who spends the most time, and therefore is most likely to form a close relationship with, the patient. In his chapter on *"Moral Perspectives"* in nursing, David Cook (1992) recognises the fact that the ethical dilemmas faced by nurses will be very familiar to other health care professionals, but adds that *". . . the nursing profession is clear that the nurse's role with regard to the patients is not exactly the same as that of the doctor. While sharing in the care of the patients, the definition of care is wider, not merely in terms of relationships but also in terms of acting on the patient's behalf as an advocate"*. There will, as Mr Cook (1992) states, be times when a patient expresses *". . . something to a nurse believing that it would go no further and yet the nurse knows that the knowledge may be relevant to the pattern of care indicated by the medical adviser. . . . Maintaining the confidentiality and trust of the patient may conflict with what may be the patient's long term interests"*. This is a problem common to all the health care professions.

The introductory clause of the UKCC (1992) code of professional conduct states that *"Each registered nurse, midwife and health visitor shall act at all times in such a manner as to safeguard and promote the interests of individual patients and clients; serve the interests of society; justify public trust and confidence and, uphold and enhance the good standing and reputation of the professions"*, indicating that a registered nursing practitioner is accountable for her actions as a professional at all times. Accountability is to the employer, but the patient's wellbeing must always be of paramount importance.

The UKCC and the GMC agree that there is a wide range of issues which call for co-operation between the professions at both a national and a local level, and endeavour to encourage this co-operation. Clause six of the UKCC (1992) code deals with collaboration and co-operation in care stating that nurses should "... *work in a collaborative and co-operative manner with health care professionals and others involved in providing care, and recognise and respect their particular contributions within the care team*", while clause five states that a nurse must make every effort to "... *work in an open and co-operative manner with patients, clients and their families, foster their independence and recognise and respect their involvement in the planning and delivery of care*".

Clause ten of the UKCC (1992) code states; "... *as a Nurse, Midwife, or Health Visitor you must* ... *protect all confidential information concerning patients and clients obtained in the course of professional practice and make disclosures only with the consent, where required by the order of a court, or where you can justify disclosure in the wider public interest*".

"*The public interest*", in the context of the UKCC (1987) advisory paper on confidentiality, covers the interests of an individual, of groups of individuals, and of society in general and is taken to include matters such as serious crime, child abuse, and drug trafficking. A nurse must "... *report to an appropriate person or authority having regard to the physical social and psychological effects on patients and clients, any circumstances in the environment of care which might jeopardise standards of practice*" and "*Report to an appropriate authority any circumstances in which safe and appropriate care for patients and clients cannot be provided*" (UKCC 1992). These reports are carried out in the patient's best interests, but may involve the communication of information to and from members of health service management.

The Council is a regulatory body and is responsible for the standards of these professions. It requires members to operate within the guidelines and, as with other statutory bodies, members can be struck off for not following their code of conduct. Collaboration and co-operation are required between those giving care and researchers. Information must only be passed on if it is seen that the purpose for which it is required is valid, if the information is only passed to persons who are bound by the same standards of confidentiality, and if the means of storage of the information is secure.

Health visitors follow the guidelines set down by the UKCC. However, Carol Robertson (1991) in her book *"Health Visiting in Practice"*, highlights specific confidentiality and access problems faced by health visitors. Firstly, Ms Robertson (1991) states that health visitors have to be particularly sensitive in their recording of information, as details about clinical and personal matters are given to them with the underlying assumption of confidentiality.

The social aspects of the profession present particular dilemmas for the health visitor. As Ms Robertson (1991) asks, *"Is the better alternative to record 'personal problem discussed' or to write nothing?"* As Kate Robinson stated in 1985, *". . . Health Visitor records are not going to tell the whole truth about the work, whatever records scheme is invented"*.

There are, however, moves afoot to make health visitor recording more explicit and more subject to review, specifically encouraging these issues to be discussed between health visitors and their managers. Difficulties are especially apparent when an employing authority requests information which may be in breach of confidentiality. It is suggested that at these times, health visitors should seek advice from the Royal College of Nursing (RCN) or the Health Visitors Association (HVA). Joan Bailey explains that, *". . . in general, it is felt that employers have no legal entitlement to confidential information and that it is therefore wrong for the nurse to provide it"* (quoted in Robertson 1991).

Peter Godber (1981) states that requests to disclose case notes in court should be contested and quotes a court of appeal decision which could protect health visitors from having to surrender them (*Gaskin* v *Liverpool County Council*, see appendix A, section 1).

Ms Robertson (1991) agrees with The Royal College of Obstetricians and Gynaecologists' assertion that a child's record card will contain not only the child's details, but also information on the mother, such as number of previous births, name of GP, age. The information noted will vary from one location to another. It is common practice for the health visitor to receive this information from the discharge slip or from the midwife.

The McClymont working party in 1983 suggested that other useful shared information could include factors such as the condition of the mother and child and some social background, useful in helping to identify families meriting extra ". . . *consideration and support*" (quoted in Robertson 1991).

One very real concern, voiced by both health visitors and the social workers with whom they work closely, is that of the risk to confidentiality and possible "*stigma*" attached to the placing of information on a shared computerised record (such as whether or not a child's name appears on the Child Protection Register). In contrast to this argument, the sharing of information between agencies has been supported by some social workers and clinicians. For example, clinicians in an Accident and Emergency department might need to know whether an injured child brought into the department on a Saturday night, by a drunken parent, is registered as being vulnerable or at risk. This information is, in practice, at present available to that clinician by means of a phonecall to the keeper of the register during office hours, or to a duty social worker out of hours, but this process can take time. The general consensus seems to be that if there is any doubt about the nature of a child's injury, the child can be kept in hospital overnight or until the information becomes available.

4.9 Obstetrics And Gynaecology

Obstetricians and Gynaecologists, as members of the medical profession, are accountable to the GMC and adopt the same principals of practice as those set down by the BMA. The Royal College of Obstetricians and Gynaecologists (RCOG), however, states that in the practice of its particular branches of medicine there are areas deemed especially sensitive, and that these are recognised as such by the 1967 Abortion Act criteria on confidentiality. Patient care may require the linkage of information about two separate patients (e.g. mother and baby). Such data also help to advance the understanding of obstetrical and neonatal problems.

The College distinguishes between the definitions of the words *"confidentiality"* and *"security"*. *"Confidentiality is the concept which prevents disclosure of information given in confidence, or of identity, unless the information is necessary for treatment prevention, medical research, or as a statutory requirement"* whereas, security *". . . concerns the mechanism of keeping any form of medical record free from the risk of unauthorised access or accidental disclosure"* (RCOG 1982). The security of the record must cover any document identifying an individual patient, any document identifying an individual even if not associated with medical details, such as hospital patient information, and any documents containing medical and clinical information but not identifying an individual, including hospital summaries or annual reports.

4.10 Professions Supplementary To Medicine

The Council for the Professions Supplementary to Medicine (CPSM) in its "Infamous Conduct Statements", outlines the establishment of ethical rules and restrictions required beyond those defined by Law. The Council sits in a judicial capacity to decide cases, but emphasises the impracticability of compiling a list of what it considers to be "infamous behaviour". Each case is considered individually and is decided on its own merits.

The infamous conduct statements cover chiropodists, dieticians, medical laboratory technicians, orthoptists, occupational therapists, physiotherapists, and radiographers, all of these professions being advised to ". . . *keep or store and disclose health information about a patient solely for the purpose of that patient's continuing care, unless there is specific evidence to the contrary*". It is considered that the clinician ". . . *who has carefully followed while practising in the UK the 'Code of Confidentiality of Personal Health Data' will not be in breach of this requirement*" (CPSM 1993).

4.11 Psychology

The British Psychological Society states that a psychologist must maintain adequate records, and take all reasonable efforts to maintain the confidentiality of information gained in the course of practice or research. He must protect the privacy of individuals or organisations on whom information is held. He must make every effort to anonymise any communicated information, gained in the course of practice or research, about individuals, organisations or participants in research, from being revealed deliberately or inadvertently without their express permission (British Psychological Society 1993).

Personally identifiable information should be communicated to others only with the express permission of the identified subjects. (As with the medical professions, this statement is subject to the best interests of recipients of treatment, participants in research and the requirements of the law). This applies unless the psychologists are working in a team, in which case they should make clear to the other members of the team the need for confidentiality of the information obtained, and the extent to which personally identifiable information may be shared.

In exceptional circumstances, and when there is sufficient information to raise serious concern about the safety of recipients of the service (or of others who might be threatened by that person's behaviour) the practitioner may take steps to inform an appropriate third party without prior consent, after first consulting with an experienced and disinterested colleague (unless delay in seeking this advice would involve significant risk to life or health).

Psychologists must take steps to ensure the confidentiality of all records and to ensure that they remain personally identifiable only as long as they are in use, ensuring that any records under the psychologist's control which are no longer in use are anonymised.

It is required that psychologists take steps to safeguard the security of any records they make, including those on computer and "... *where they have limited control over access, exercise discretion over the information entered on the record*" (British Psychological Society 1993).

4.12 Non Medical Staff

The MPS advises that doctors should ensure that all members of a health care team are aware of the ethics principle and are constantly mindful of it. Case notes should be kept securely and access should be controlled most strictly. It is the clinician who is in charge of the patient's care and is therefore ethically responsible for the confidentiality of the medical record. This should not be overlooked even if that responsibility is delegated, for example, to a medical records officer. The different members of the team (e.g. a social worker, or a home help) may have different loyalties, and a doctor should exercise some caution when asked to participate in case conferences.

Similarly, the UKCC states that it is advisable that the contracts of employment of all employees not directly involved with the patients/clients, but having access to or handling confidential records, contain clauses which emphasise the principles of confidentiality, and state the disciplinary consequences of breaching them. Paragraph 3.20 of the report from the Confidentiality Working Group of the DHSS Steering Group on Health Services Information, suggests a form of words worthy of consideration as follows:

> *"In the course of your duties you may have access to confidential material about patients, members of staff or other health service business. On no account must information relating to identifiable patients be divulged to anyone other than authorised persons for example medical, nursing or other professional staff as appropriate who are concerned directly with the care, diagnosis and or treatment of the patient. If you are in any doubt whatsoever as to the authority of a person or body asking for information of this nature you must seek advice from your superior officer. Similarly, no information of a personal or confidential nature concerning individual members of staff should be divulged to anyone without the proper authority having first been given. Failure to observe these rules will be regarded by your employer as serious and will result in disciplinary action being taken against you, including dismissal"* (Körner 1984).

The Royal College of Obstetricians and Gynaecologists states that each hospital or clinic holding records, should have a written code of practice formulated by the organisation, under the guidance of the Local Ethics Committee or Privacy Committee (RCOG 1982). These codes of practice should be familiar to all staff who may, in the course of their duty, have cause to handle medical files at any time during or after a patient's course of treatment. These would include (for instance) medical records staff, hospital social workers, porters, domestic staff, drivers and computer staff. The code of practice should be safeguarded by agreed sanctions.

The BMA and GMC both state that, ethically, doctors carry primary responsibility for the protection of information obtained in the course of treating a patient, and are subsequently responsible for ensuring the security and confidentiality of manual and computerised records. However, the common law position, as reflected in the Department of Health's policies and procedures, states that the body holding the record is ultimately responsible for any decisions made about the disclosure of information from that record and, subsequently, the processing of that information.

The duty of confidentiality also lies with those who receive information indirectly in the course of non-clinical and administrative duties with health authorities, commercial firms, insurance companies, local authorities and the pharmaceutical industry. The MPS maintains that journalism and authorship should be included in this statement.

5.1 Disclosure To Health Service Management

Concern has arisen recently over the safeguarding of confidential patient information which might appear, for example, on bills for extra-contractual referrals. The BMA (1992) quote the IMG (1990) thus, *"Very strict, tightly controlled administrative and computer security arrangements will be necessary to safeguard confidentiality and to deal with subject access requests"*. The BMA (1992) also says that *". . . all NHS staff should be made aware . . . that breach of confidence is a disciplinary offence and arrangements for handling data containing patient's details must be agreed with an appropriate senior medical officer"*.

The GMC distinguishes between administrative staff who are directly involved with patient care, e.g. secretaries who type referral letters, and staff whose work is not of direct benefit to the patient, e.g. those involved in research, education and audit. In the latter case patients should be given the opportunity to withhold their consent to disclosure.

5.1.1 Audit

One of the main purposes of medical and clinical audit is that through the study of individual patient records, and the linking of information around the treatment of that individual, it is possible to establish outcome measures (Rigby et al 1992). It is therefore inevitable that in some cases an individual will have to be identified for the links to be established, although it is possible to conduct medical audit without using patient names. As the Conference of the Royal Medical and Surgical Colleges of Great Britain and Northern Ireland points out, there is a potential conflict of interest between the data requirements of medical audit and the needs of patients and practitioners for confidentiality (Conference of Medical Royal Colleges and their faculties in the UK 1991).

Staff handling the information *". . . who will normally be led by a medical practitioner"* (Department of Health 1991) must be made aware of the importance and sensitivity of the records, and are under an obligation to treat the records with the same care as the original record holder. Also, to try and minimise the risk of a breach of confidentiality, it is good practice that *"at the earliest opportunity, explicit patient identifiers should be removed from the record in favour of secondary identifiers such as NHS number or PAS number"* (Rigby et al 1992).

The results of the audit, as the Conference of Colleges states, must only show aggregated information and general conclusions, so that they can be passed to management and Health Authorities without compromising the individual's right of anonymity. The reports should cover the general areas of activity audited, the overall conclusions made, and the plans for action or procedural change. There should also be a record made of the review of any resulting changes. In addition, all written or computerised records of audit meetings must be totally anonymised, with working protocols and proforma not being kept, as these duplicate information already available in the primary medical record (Network 1992). In practice, however, most cases discussed at an audit review meeting (e.g. in a monthly perinatal mortality meeting), are so specialised, and occur so infrequently, that most staff will already be aware of the identity of the individual patients.

5.2   Research

The commonest areas in which issues of confidentiality are raised with regard to research are:

- research based solely on clinical records
- research involving contact with patients
- research involving children, mentally incapacitated or comatose patients, and
- research involving subjects identified not from clinical records but in some other way.

The way in which research is carried out varies from study to study. Common to all is the role of the Local Research Ethics Committees (LREC). The LRECs are district-based, and are responsible for looking after the interests of patients who are involved in clinical research studies. The committee must be satisfied that each project:

(a)   has been properly assessed to establish the scientific merit

(b)   is properly supervised

(c)   is safe, and no discomfort or distress will be caused to the participants

(d)   will not adversely affect the state of health of the participants

(e)   recruits participants lawfully, and permits them to freely drop out of the study

(f)   maintains confidentiality, and

(g)   offers no improper financial inducements to researchers or participants.

Although the LRECs oversee the projects, responsibility for the security and proper use of health information still ultimately rests with the named doctor, dental practitioner, nurse or other health care practitioner leading the research (Rigby et al 1992). In the rare cases where a registered practitioner is not involved, a suitable person must be chosen for this role. That practitioner is then responsible for ensuring that all staff who handle research information adhere to the rules for maintaining confidentiality of personal information, and sign a declaration of confidentiality as part of their written contract of employment.

The BMA, GMC, and MPS all agree that it is ethical to disclose information for the purpose of medical research which has been approved by an LREC. The British Society of Gynaecologists and Obstetricians states that access to information for clinical research ". . . *is essential but can only be released to a bona fide research worker with the permission of the consultant involved in the treat-*

ment of the case or if this is not possible with the permission of an independent ethical or privacy committee" (quoted in Rigby et al 1992).

The final results of the research must be published in a manner that ensures that the identification or partial identification of the people or groups involved is impossible.

Situations unique to the types of research identified at the top of section 5.2 are covered in the following paragraphs.

5.2.1 Research Based Solely on Health Care Records

Consent to carry out this type of research must be sought by the researcher from the record holder. The patient's express permission does not need to be obtained. The LREC should be consulted in cases of doubt.

5.2.2 Research which Involves Contact with Patients

A health care researcher who wishes to approach a potential participant identified from the health record, must first approach the record holder to explain the purpose and nature of the study. The record holder or the researcher (depending on the course of action decided upon) may then approach the patient, making sure that he has notice and full details of the proposed visit, and a detailed description of how and why he has been selected. The patient must be made fully aware of the absolute right, at any stage of the process, to withdraw from or refuse to participate in any form of research.

Ethical responsibilities and considerations should be seriously considered when the research involves invasive procedures, such as physical examination. Department of Health policy states that the body with responsibility for the record also has responsibility for contacting the patient before any information is disclosed to the researcher.

5.2.3 Research Involving Children, Mentally Incapacitated, or Comatose Patients

Researchers have a special responsibility to ensure that these groups are protected from harm or distress. Consent to gather information for research purposes should be sought from parents, guardians, or doctors acting in respect of detained patients, or from another appropriate authority. This view is put forward by the MRC (1985), but the MPS challenges it, citing a case, on the basis that no one can give consent for mentally handicapped or mentally ill people. In the case of mental incapacity, information gathering for research purposes may need to proceed without specific consent. This is only acceptable where the individual receiving care is unable to give consent and where there is no close contact with relatives. Those who proceed without consent in these circumstances must be satisfied that the activity is ". . . *directed to the provision of appropriate or improved services for future recipients of care*" (MRC 1985). It can be assumed that this would mean in practice that aggregated information would not adversely affect the patient and therefore could be communicated for the planning of future services, and hopefully the future benefit of others.

5.2.3.1 Consent for Research on Children

In its guidelines on research, the British Paediatric Association (BPA) states that legally valid consent should be obtained, where possible from the child, or from the parent, or guardian as appropriate (BPA Ethics Advisory Committee 1992). Children are unique under English law as they are the only group on whose behalf other individuals may automatically give consent for medical procedures. There is division of legal opinion as to whether or not a parent or guardian may give legally valid consent for a non-therapeutic procedure or for pure research on children. In addition, children are less able to challenge records about themselves, and have more years to suffer any adverse reactions from research. As the BPA (1992) states in its guidelines, *"This partnership should accord with the declaration of Helsinki, in that concern for the interests of the subject must always prevail over those of science and society".*

5.2.4 Research Involving Patients Not Identified by Health Care Records

The subjects involved in this type of research are individuals who are not patients in the context of the matter under investigation. Most often they are either the members of a control group against which the "cases" are to be compared, or are the (usually randomly selected) subjects of a survey. They are entitled to the same protection from harm and embarrassment as persons participating in any type of medical study. Explicit consent must be given by the participant and the local LREC, but in this instance need not be sought from the General Practitioner.

5.3 Teaching

For both undergraduate and postgraduate teaching, the GMC (1993) states that *"Where disclosure would enable one or more individuals to be identified, the patients concerned, or those who may properly give permission on their behalf, must wherever possible be made aware of that possibility and be advised that they may at any stage withhold their consent to disclosure".*

The GMC states that disclosure in the public interest is rarely justifiable, but examples would include instances where the non-disclosure of information would expose the patient, or someone else, to the risk of death or serious harm. In the words of the BMA (1992) *"The patient's right to confidence is qualified, not absolute"*. The MPS states that there will sometimes be a conflict between the best interests of the patient and the dictates of the doctor's own conscience, and suggests that at these times, the doctor should consult with colleagues. Some practical problems might include the following.

6.1 AIDS and HIV

Neither positive HIV nor AIDS is a statutorily notifiable condition, and therefore the usual ethical considerations apply. Hospital employees are under an obligation not to disclose the identity of AIDS patients, this duty being upheld by the British courts. The case of *X* v *Y* [10] in 1988, gives clear legal authority in support of the preservation of confidentiality to AIDS patients (including those health care professionals who suffer from the disease) and it does so in the public interest. The BMA (1992) in its book, *"The Rights and Responsibilities of Doctors"*, recognises that the disclosure of information regarding a person's HIV status could have a serious effect on both the psychological and social well-being of the patient, and his livelihood, accommodation and relationships. If people are to come forward for testing, counselling and treatment, confidentiality must not be breached. On the other hand the doctor may feel that there is a public interest argument in disclosing the HIV status of a person to people who may be at risk of infection.

The GMC (1993) guidance on HIV and AIDS states that: *"If the patient refuses consent for the general practitioner to be told [about the patients infection], then the doctor has two sets of obligations to*

---

[10][1988] 2 All ER 648

consider: obligations to the patient to maintain confidence, and obligations to other carers whose own health may be put unnecessarily at risk. In such circumstances the patient should be counselled about the difficulties which his or her condition is likely to pose for the team responsible for providing continuing health care and about the likely consequences for the standard of care which can be provided in the future. If, having considered the matter carefully in the light of such counselling, the patient still refuses to allow the general practitioner to be informed then the patient's request for privacy should be respected. The only exception to that general principle arises where the doctor judges that the failure to disclose would put the health of any of the health care team at risk. The Council believes that, in such a situation, it would not be improper to disclose such information as that person needs to know."

6.2 Child Protection

In child protection work, *"the needs of the children must always be regarded [by clinicians] as of first importance as their age and vulnerability renders them powerless to protect their own interests"* (Joint Working Party of DoH et al 1993). In situations where a doctor suspects that a patient may be the victim of abuse, the GMC (1993) states that *"In such circumstances the patient's interests are paramount and will usually require the doctor to disclose relevant information to an appropriate, responsible person or an officer of a statutory agency"*.

A clinician's first duty being to the child, other parties involved in a particular case, e.g. the child's parents, *"should be made aware that information will be shared on a controlled 'need to know' basis in the interests of the child"* (Joint Working Party of DoH et al 1993). These exceptional circumstances do not however absolve a clinician from his duty of confidentiality. It requires a balanced judgement to be made between the justification for breaching confidence and the distress that this will cause, and the withholding

of potentially vital information obtained within the privileged
doctor-patient relationship.

The Department of Health is in the process of revising its guidelines on child protection. They should become available during
1994.

6.3 The DVLA

The duty to notify the DVLA about medical conditions rests with
the patient. If the doctor discovers that a patient is driving, having
been deemed unfit to do so, he may warn the patient, noting the
warning in his record. If the patient carries on driving, it may then
be ethical, according to the MPS, for the doctor to notify the DVLA.

6.4 Police Requests For Information

The general position is that it is not a criminal offence not to reveal
information to the police about a crime. In the case of *Rice* v
Connolly[11] cited by the BMA (1992), Lord Justice Parker stated:
*"It seems to me quite clear that though every citizen has a moral
duty or, if you like, a social duty to assist the police, there is no legal
duty to that effect"*.

When asked for information by the police, it is often best in the
first instance to ask for proof of the patient's permission. When the
patient is not aware of an enquiry, it is left to the doctor's discretion. There are, however, certain statutes which require that a
person should answer certain questions asked by the police and it
is agreed that a doctor is not exempt from this requirement because
he believes the information to be confidential. For example, the
BMA cites another case, *Hunter* v *Mann*[12] where the court found
that *"... a doctor is not exempt from the statutory obligation under*

---

[11][1966] 2 QB 414, [1966] 2 All ER 649   [12][1974] 2 All ER 414

the Road Traffic Act, to supply information about the identity of people injured in a road accident" (BMA 1992).

6.5 During Court Proceedings

A doctor can be summoned to attend a Coroner, Procurator Fiscal, Judge, or similar officer of the court. Information should not be disclosed by a doctor in response to demands from a third party solicitor or court official. Information may be disclosed to the chairman of a committee investigating a practitioner's fitness to practice, provided that every reasonable effort has been made to seek the patient's consent.

6.6 In Cases Involving Treason

Doctors may in the course of their practice become privileged to confidential information which may or may not be related to a person's health, but which could be important evidence in a case of treason. It is an offence in English law for a person who believes that another has committed treason not to disclose information to the authorities.

7.1 Disclosure Of Information To The Patient

The BMA states that the secrets are those of the patient, and therefore the doctor has an obligation to disclose information to the patient or to his legal advisor. In contrast to this statement, both the GMC and the MPS put forward the view that the doctor should at all times protect the best interests of the patient. If in doing so he or she believes, and can justify the assertion, that information may be detrimental to a patient's mental or physical health (or to that of another individual) the patient can be refused access. In addition, in exceptional circumstances, and when it is in the patients best medical interests to do so, it is deemed acceptable for a doctor to divulge some items of information to some other people. The Data Protection Act 1984 supports this argument with a clause stating that medical records are subject to special exemptions under the Act.

The nursing profession can at times be faced with the question of how much a patient should be told about his or her own medical condition. Especially bearing in mind the more day-to-day nature of the nurse's relationship with a patient, the authors state in *"Managing Nursing Work"*, that *"While there may be a strong belief in sharing information with patients, sensitivity to those who do not wish for more knowledge must be respected"* (Vaughan & Pillmore 1989).

7.2 Disclosure Of Information To Relatives And To Third Parties

The MPS states that on occasions when it is undesirable on medical grounds to seek the consent of the patient, the doctor may give information in confidence to a relative or other appropriate person, when this is in the best medical interests of the patient. Similarly, if the doctor feels that the disclosure of information to a third party is in the patient's best interests, he can try and persuade the patient to give consent to that disclosure. When the patient has refused, the doctor may only then disclose that information in the most extreme circumstances.

The right of parents to have access to the·health records of their children raises problems for many paediatricians. Such records, especially in cases of child abuse or suspected child abuse, include opinion, deduction, and surmise, as well as facts which it would at times not be in the child's best interests for the parents to see. However, it is becoming increasingly common for the parents to hold their child's own health record, which requires skillful handling by all concerned.

In practice, the nursing profession, especially in the community, may be more willing and indeed may have more reason to divulge medical information to members of the patient's family. The activities of the family (and sometimes of close friends) are often an integral part of the care package given, or care plan constructed.

References to Chapters 3 to 7

British Medical Association. 1993. *Confidentiality & People Under 16, Guidance issued jointly by the BMA, GMSC, HEA, Brook Advisory Centres, FPA and RCGP*. BMA.

British Medical Association Professional Division. 1992. *Rights and Responsibilities of Doctors*. 2nd ed. Tavistock Square, London: BMJ Publishing Group.

British Paediatric Association Ethics Advisory Committee. August 1992. *Guidelines for the Ethical Conduct of Medical Research Involving Children*. London: BPA.

British Psychological Society. April 1993. *Code of Conduct, Ethical Principles & Guidelines*. Leicester: BPS.

Conference of Medical Royal Colleges and their Faculties in the United Kingdom. Interim Guidelines on Confidentiality and Medical Audit. 14th December 1991. *British Medical Journal*, Vol. 303, p. 1525.

Cook D. 1992. Moral Perspectives. In *Knowledge for Nursing Practice*. Robinson, K. & Vaughan, B. (Editors). Oxford: Butterworth-Heinemann.

Council for Professions Supplementary to Medicine. August and October 1993. *Infamous Conduct Statements*. London: CPSM.

Department of Health. January 1991. *Assuring The Quality Of Medical Care: Implementation Of Medical & Dental Audit In The Hospital And Community Health Services*. HC(91)2.

Department of Health, Information Management Group. 1990. *NHS Review, Information Systems: Action for Managers*. London: DoH.

General Medical Council. May 1993. *HIV Infection and AIDS: The Ethical Considerations*. London: GMC.

General Medical Council. December 1993. *Professional Conduct And Discipline: Fitness To Practise*. London: GMC.

Godber, P. May 1981. Confidentiality Of Case Records. *Health Visitor*, Vol. 54, p. 193.

Joint Working Party of the Department of Health, British Medical Association and Conference of Medical Royal Colleges. November 1993. *Child Protection: Medical Responsibilities*.

Körner, E. October 1984. *The Protection and Maintenance of Confidentiality of Patient and Employee Data. A Report From The Confidentiality Working Group*. Steering Group on Health Services Information. HMSO: London.

Medical Research Council. 1985. *Responsibility In The Use Of Personal Information For Research*. London: MRC.

Medical Protection Society. 1992. *Disclosure Of Medical Records*. London: MPS.

Rigby, M., McBride, A. & Shiels, C. 1992. *Computers In Medical Audit*, 2nd ed. London: Royal Society of Medicine.

Robertson, C. 1991. *Health Visiting In Practice*, 2nd ed. Edinburgh: Churchill Livingstone.

Robinson, K. 1985. Knowledge and its relationship to health visiting, in *Health Visiting*. Luker, K. and Orr, J. (Editors). Oxford: Blackwell.

Royal College Of Obstetricians And Gynaecologists. November 1982. *Statement On Confidentiality*. London: RCOG.

United Kingdom Central Council for Nursing, Midwifery and Health Visiting. June 1992. *Code Of Professional Conduct*. London: UKCC.

United Kingdom Central Council for Nursing, Midwifery and Health Visiting. April 1987. *Confidentiality: An Elaboration Of Clause 9 Of The Second Edition Of The UKCC's Code Of Professional Conduct For The Nurse, Midwife and Health Visitor*. London: UKCC.

Vaughan, B. & Pillmore, M. (Editors). 1989. *Managing Nursing Work*. London: Scutari Press.

Case Law

The three cases below illustrate the legal position on the confidentiality of medical information. The first case involves Liverpool City Council's refusal to disclose information in court in 1980, the second describes *Gillick v Norfolk and Wisbech AHA* concerning the relationship between parents and children, the third relates to Mid-Glamorgan Health Authority's refusal to disclose a medical record to the patient. All of the rulings concluded that information is confidential and that a patient or court has no common law right of access to medical information.

1 Gaskin v Liverpool City Council 1980[13]

The Appeal court ruled in this case that *"child care officers should not be compelled to produce . . ."* in court confidential records about a child that the officer had made while looking after the child. As a result Liverpool City Council were not forced to produce reports, files, and case notes made by social workers and others who had been looking after the child. The judges stated that *"it was necessary for the proper functioning of the child care service that the confidentiality of the relevant documents should be preserved"*.

As a result, practitioners looking after children, when asked to appear in court proceedings and to produce case records, should seek legal advice with a view to contesting such a request, on the grounds that the professional's notes are confidential and, in legal terms, privileged (Godber 1981).

2 Gillick v Norfolk And Wisbech Area Health Authority 1985

This House of Lords ruling concerned the relationship between parents and children. Ms Gillick wanted an assurance from the Health Authority that her daughters, while under the age of

---

[13][1980] 1 WLR 1549 CA.

consent, would only receive contraceptive advice and treatment with her consent.

Lord Scarman presiding over the case, acknowledged that parents do have rights, but only as long as these rights are exercised in the protection of the child's person or property. He went on to state that *"parental rights yield to the child's right to make his own decisions when he reaches a sufficient understanding and intelligence to be capable of making up his own mind on the matter requiring decision"* (BMA 1992).

The ruling of the case established that a young person who is able to fully understand what is proposed and its implications (in the doctor's opinion), is competent to consent to medical treatment, regardless of age (BMA 1993).

3 R v Mid-Glamorgan Family Health Services Authority 1993[14]

The background to the case was that the applicant had suffered depression and psychological problems since 1966, and had asked the FHSA for access to his medical records for information about his past and formative years. This request was turned down, as was a further request by the applicant to Mid-Glamorgan Health Authority (who would have considered disclosure on the condition that no potential litigation was contemplated by the applicant). Both respondents had offered disclosure to a medical adviser nominated by the applicant, but this offer was declined by the applicant.

The applicant argued that the refusal to disclose involved a denial of respect for a person's private life, and that a patient of sound mind had a right to receive all relevant information which he sought.

---

[14][1993] 137 SJ 153.

Mr Justice Popplewell presiding over the case stated that neither the Data Protection Act 1984, nor the Access to Health Records Act 1990 were of relevance in this case, because the records in question pre-dated these pieces of legislation. However, it was submitted that since a patient had the right to receive relevant information prior to making a decision about treatment, he had a right to understand after treatment what treatment he had received. There might of course be a difference between the doctor generally explaining what had happened and the patient being provided with the detailed written records which were never intended for his eyes. It was also stated that the opinion of a doctor was his alone, and the fact that the patient provided the information was irrelevant, and therefore did not entitle him to see the conclusions of the doctor based on that information.

It was concluded that even if the applicant did have some rights of access to his medical records, these were conditional, and the respondents had offered all that was necessary to comply with their duty to the applicant (Ying Hui Tan 1993).

References

British Medical Association. 1992. *Rights And Responsibilities Of Doctors*. London: BMJ Publishing Group.

British Medical Association. 1993. *Confidentiality & People Under 16*. London: BMA.

Godber, P. May 1981. Confidentiality Of Case Records. *Health Visitor*, Vol. 54, p. 193.

Ying Hui Tan, 8 June 1993. No Right Of Access To Health Records, Law Report. *Independent Newspaper*.

Social Care Guidelines

1 What Do They Need To Know?

It is universally agreed that social workers and other staff connected with the social services care of an individual, do at times require some information about the personal health of that individual. It is also accepted that social workers need to pass on information which they have collected to health care professionals for the purposes of the health or social care of that individual. However, it is also agreed that there are both formal and informal restrictions on the transfer of information between the social services, the health authorities and some other bodies, whether done by computer, on paper or by word of mouth.

From the computer transfer point of view, Michael Cross in an article in the Health Service Journal (1993) stated that in placing personal and health information on computer, ". . . *Networking enthusiasts face . . . [their] worst nightmare along the way. This is the need to bring local authority community health records onto the network. 'Most places will probably have that problem filed under 'too difficult to think about''*, says one computer executive".

Some examples of a need to share information between health professionals and social services staff follow:

(a) The Child Protection Register, is kept by an officer of the Local Authority, but is important to health visitors, GP's and clinicians in Accident and Emergency departments. Generally, in cases of child abuse, information needs to be exchanged in the interests of the child.

(b) Meals on wheels services, the need for which is assessed by social workers, but which have people referred to them by health care professionals.

(c)   Home helps, another service assessed by social workers which complements the provision of health services.

(d)   Occupational therapists are often employed by the Local Authority and have health care training as well as counselling and assessment skills. Dealing with the physically handicapped, they must have some information about the health of their client. A barrier to sharing information would be the fact that they are providing a service for which there is an assessment procedure and the possibility of refusal (e.g. assistance with physical aids or the supply of disabled drivers badges). This is a problem with many of the services provided by the Social Services, but is especially pronounced in occupational therapy.

(e)   Community mental handicap teams which contain staff from both health and social care services.

(f)   Communications between community psychiatric nurses and psychiatric social workers.

(g)   Communications between child care teams and health visitors.

(h)   Case conferences which provide a forum for sharing both social and health care information between health professionals, social workers, other external bodies and individual carers.

2 Principles Of The British Association Of Social Workers

The eleventh principle of the British Association of Social Workers' (BASW 1986) code of ethics states that members should always ensure:

> *"Confidentiality of information and divulgence only by consent or exceptionally in evidence of serious danger."*

The code then goes on to state that:

> ". . . *the multi-purpose agency, in particular has to consider what arrangements should be made to guard against the misuse of information. The paper on confidentiality, {produced by the BASW} after outlining situations in which the client's right to confidentiality might be over-ridden, states: 'in all the foregoing circumstances the breach of confidence must remain limited to the needs of the situation at that time and in no circumstances can the worker assume a carte blanche to reveal matters which are not relevant to a situation'.*" (BASW 1986)

The eighth principle states that a BASW member must operate a system of:

> "*collaboration with others in the interests of clients*", recognising the need to collaborate with others ". . . *in the interests of their clients*", and placing the obligation upon social workers not only to be alert to that need, but also to take any necessary or appropriate action (BASW 1986).

3 The Access To Personal Files Act 1987, And The Access To Personal Files (Social Services) Regulations 1989 - Who Has Right Of Access?

The Access To Personal Files Act 1987 gives the right of access to files by any user of the Social Services, and by any other living person about whom an Authority holds "*accessible personal information*" in order to carry out Social Service functions (as defined by the Local Authority Social Services Act 1970). Where a composite file is maintained for an Authority's dealings with a family, each member of that composite group, for example a family member, has the right of access to information about him, but not to that of any other member of his family without consent.

The Act does not confer a right of access upon the staff of a Local Authority to information about themselves, which is held for management purposes rather than for an Authority's Social Services function. Should a member of staff also be in receipt of Social Services care, the individual in question should have the same rights as any other user in his capacity as a user of those services. The exceptions to the first rule are foster parents, those Registered under the Registered Homes Act 1984 as amended by the Registered Homes (Amendment) Act 1991, and other carers who are not employees of the Local Authority who would have the right of access to information about themselves. This legislation does not apply to the records of a voluntary agency, or other bodies, even if they are acting as the agent of a Local Authority.

4 Personal Information - A Definition

"Personal information" is information about a living individual who can be identified either from the information itself, or from that and other information in the possession of the holder. Personal information includes the expression of an opinion about a person, but not any indication of the intention of an authority towards him. However, this does not prevent the Authority from letting another individual know what their intentions are towards the client. Generally, clients are informed of an Authority's intentions in the course of continuing care. This is seen as part of the process of encouraging service users to participate as far as possible in actions concerning them.

Information includes that held in files, card indexes and day books, and that prepared and held by Social Services departments in connection with judicial proceedings. This information may be held in area offices and in other Social Service Establishments such as residential homes and by hospital social workers employed by the Local Authority.

Information recorded before the Regulations came into force is not covered unless earlier information is needed to make sense of that recorded after the enforcement of the regulations.

5 Shared Files

A circular issued by the Welsh Office in February 1989 stated that
there are already existing protocols for joint working and joint
record keeping between the Local Authority and other organisations. These include child guidance and community mental health
teams. In the case of shared files, the Authority must first decide
whether the information is covered by the provisions of the Regulations, after considering the details of the arrangements in each
case. In addition, where a joint record is kept between the Social
Services and another department of the Local Authority, the
information recorded in a file kept by a staff member of the Social
Services department would be subject to these Regulations.

6 Information Relating To Another Individual

Information relating to a third party is often held within an
individual's file. This may refer either to (a) information about the
third party, or (b) what the third party has said, either about the
individual or about someone else. Information of this type should
not be released without the consent of the parties concerned.

- In situation (a), the third party must agree to disclosure to the
  individual, and both these parties must agree to wider disclosure.
- In situation (b) the third party must agree to disclosure of the
  information to the individual.

These rules should apply, even where this may cause problems
in knowing how to allow only limited parts of the file to be disclosed.

The Regulations recognise the ability of the Authority to exercise the
use of common sense and allow for information to sometimes be
given without the express consent of an individual. An example of
this is where the individual has referred to, spoken of, or given the
other information in the first place.

7 Editing Of Information To Protect Identity

In editing information to protect an individual's identity the minimum amount of alteration should be made. An example of an acceptable change would be the omission of a name from a sentence and its replacement with an X.

8 Protection Of The Identity Of Staff Members

The Regulations do not enable an Authority to deny access where the other person whose identity would be disclosed is one who:

(a)   is or has been employed by an Authority in pursuance of its Social Services function

or

(b)   has performed for reward received direct from an Authority, a Social Services or similar function. Examples might include foster parents, child minders or informal carers who have received payment, but does not include those who do the work on a voluntary basis. A person who is merely reimbursed expenses by the authority may have his identity protected.

The Authority may therefore protect the identity of a person who it does not employ for its Social Services functions, but may not protect the identity of any of its employees carrying out a Social Services function. On occasions where the two roles overlap (e.g. a carer might, at the same time, act in more than one capacity, say as an unpaid foster parent and as a child minder paid by the Local Authority), the question of whether or not the individual's identity needs to be protected will be answered depending on the capacity in which the information was given.

This rule applies only to that information which was given in a formal capacity, or in connection with the performance of the function.

9 Capacity To Understand A Request

Where the Authority believes that the child making the request for access is capable of understanding the nature of that request, the reply must be made directly to that child. The child's application should be in writing, but does not have to be in a set format.

The Authority may either interview the child in order to satisfy itself that he is fully capable of understanding the nature of the request, or in the case of a postal request, may contact the parent or other adult. These precautions are not necessary when the Authority already has evidence in its possession that the child has sufficient capacity to understand the meaning and implications of an application. The capacity of a child to make an informed request should not be determined by a set age limit.

10 Applications By Parents

Where the Authority has reason to believe that the child does not understand, the parent (or person with legal authority to act on that child's behalf), has the right to make an application, and to receive the reply. Where an application is made by a parent in respect of a child's file, the parent must satisfy the Authority either that the child has instructed that parent to apply for access, or that the child has insufficient understanding of what an application entails, and lacks the capacity to apply in his or her own right.

The validity of the declaration should be accepted unless there are grounds to believe that the child is able to understand, or might not give consent for, the parents to have access to his file. In these circumstances, the Authority should make further enquiries as appropriate. The Authority is responsible for endeavouring to ensure that a request for access by a parent on behalf of a child is a valid request, and is done in the interests of the child, and not the parent.

11 People With Mental Disorders

No specific provision is made in the Access to Personal Files (Social Services) Regulations 1989. Applications on behalf of those who are not able to manage their own affairs because of a mental disorder can be made by a person acting under a court order, or acting within the terms of an enduring power of attorney. If the person is under 18, the regulations regarding children apply. Otherwise, the request must be made through an agent for access to the record or file. An Authority is obliged to reply to a request for information if it is satisfied that the individual has authorised the agent to make the request. The agent is responsible for providing evidence to that effect.

12 Access To A File Through An Agent

Any person of sound mind may apply for access to his file using an agent. It is up to the agent to satisfy the Authority that his authorization to gain access to a file is a valid one.

13 Exemptions

13.1 Exemptions In Respect Of Children's Files

An exemption from disclosure covers damage to the child's physical, mental or emotional state, and restricts a child's access to see his file. At times, it may also be considered that granting access to a parent on behalf of a child may be damaging to his physical or mental health, emotional wellbeing, or development. In such cases, the Authority can apply the exemption that applies to such risks.

13.2 Serious Harm

When there is reasonable cause to believe that access to the information included in a file might result in serious harm to the client's physical health, mental health or emotional condition, or to that of some other person, including a member of the Social Services staff, access to information in a file can be refused. When considering what might be covered by the term "serious harm", the guidance states that it is important to remember the fundamental principle of the right of a person to see what is written about him which, after all, forms the basis for this act.

> *"The Authority may only withhold just so much of the informa- tion which is likely to cause serious harm. It is envisaged that withholding information on this ground would be most exceptional."* (Welsh Office 1989)

However, it is recognised that the risk of child abuse, neglect or where the individual has a mental disorder, would come under this umbrella.

> *"A minority who are unstable, or have little insight may excep- tionally need to be protected permanently from certain damag- ing revelations about themselves, which might otherwise cause serious harm to themselves or cause them to act in a way that could cause serious harm to another person."* (Welsh Office 1989)

13.3 Prevention Of Crime

Information held for the purposes of the detection of crime or the apprehension or prosecution of offenders is exempt from access, if access to the information held would be likely to prejudice one of these purposes. This applies not only to information originated by the Authority itself, but also to that received from another organi- sation, such as the police.

13.4 Legal Professional Privilege

> *"Personal information is exempt from access if it consists of information in respect of which a claim to legal professional privilege would be maintained in legal proceedings."* (Welsh Office 1989)

Where the information contains some advice given by the Authority's lawyers, those lawyers should be consulted as to whether or not the access should be given.

14 Information From Health Professionals

The term "health professional", for the purposes of these regulations, includes those listed below:

Registered Medical Practitioner - Medical Act 1983 Section 55

Registered Dentist - Dentists Act 1984 Section 53(1)

Registered Optician - Opticians Act 1958 Section 30(1)

Registered Pharmaceutical Chemist - Pharmacy Act 1954 Section 24(1)

Registered Nurse, Midwife or Health Visitor - Nurses, Midwives and Health Visitors Act 1979

Registered Chiropodist, Dietician, Occupational Therapist, Orthoptist or Physiotherapist - Professions Supplementary to Medicine Act 1979

Clinical Psychologist, Child Psychotherapist or Speech Therapist

Art Therapist or Music Therapist employed by a Health Authority

Scientist Employed by such an Authority as a Head of Department

15 Personal Health Information

There is a distinction to be made between two types of personal health information:

(a)   information supplied by, or on behalf of, a "health professional", acting in a professional capacity
and

(b)   information about a person's health generated in some other way e.g. by the staff of the Social Service department themselves, or another department of the Local Authority.

15.1 Requests For Personal Health Information

A request might be made by an individual for access to personal health information held on Social Services files. Where this occurs, the "appropriate health professional" should be asked whether all the information can be disclosed, whether only part of the information can be disclosed, or whether there is a disclosure exemption on all of that information. The term "appropriate health professional" is defined as ". . . *the medical or dental practitioner who is currently, or was most recently responsible for the clinical care of that individual in connection with the matters to which the information which is the subject of the request relates.*" (Welsh Office 1989)

Where the information has come from a health professional in the course of his employment with a Health Authority, the Local Authority should direct the correspondence to the Health Authority who will then contact the "appropriate health professional" for a decision. Where the information came from another health professional, for example, a GP, the Local Authority should write to the health professional himself. The Local Authority in these cases should point out that in the absence of a response within the time limit, it is obliged to provide access. The Local Authority is obliged to abide by the decision of the health care professional. The Authority should advise its users who require or wish to seek explanation or amplification of personal health information, to discuss the matter with the *"appropriate health professional"*.

15.2 Withholding Personal Health Information
Information can be withheld because of the risk of serious harm, or withheld or edited so as not to reveal the identity of another person without consent.

15.3 Procedures
Authorities are advised to ensure that their procedures include mechanisms for:

> (a)   the appointment of a member of senior management to oversee and ensure that the regulations are adhered to in respect of

(i)   the withholding of information, and

(ii) liaison between the Local Authority and the Health Authorities, and health professionals

(b)   dealing with the validity of a child's, or his parent's, request for access

(c)   "joint working arrangements".

A Department of Health circular issued to all Social Services Directors and County Councils for action, and Community Health Councils and Health Authorities for information, in September 1988 advises that, in deciding whether to withhold information, the advice of the Authority's lawyers should normally be sought. It also advises that a record should be kept of the instances where a Local Authority has felt it necessary for information to be withheld, because of the risk of serious harm to the physical or mental health, or emotional condition of an individual, or that of another person.

15.4 Information From Health Professionals Given To Social Services

Health professionals are under an obligation to protect health care information in their possession, and to ensure that it is treated with the same respect by all those who might come into contact with it. Social Services staff must ensure that:

(a)   the information is used only for the purposes for which that information was disclosed

(b)   it is not passed to anyone unless for that purpose

(c)   the information received will not be passed on to a third party without the agreement of the health professional.

In summary, personal health information given to Social Services staff by a health professional can only be disclosed:

(a)   in compliance with a court order

(b)   in compliance with a statutory requirement

(c)   so that health care can be provided to a client or patient for the purposes of their care.

"If further disclosure is proposed for a purpose associated with the provision of health care then the appropriate health professional must be consulted and his consent obtained."
(DoH 1988)

It is recognised as vital that, in the course of providing care, Health Authorities and Social Services should co operate; the effectiveness of that care being based on the free and unhampered flow of information between them.

16 The General Principles Of Confidentiality And Access Within The Social Services And The Local Authority

16.1 Other Personal Information
The term "other personal information" covers personal information held on file, excluding personal health information which has been received from a health professional.

16.2 The General Principle
The general principle is that all information should be regarded as confidential and that information can only be disclosed without the consent of the subject for the following reasons, and on the following occasions.

16.2.1 Local Authority Staff in Contact with Social Services
The duty of confidentiality should be noted in the conditions of service of all Local Authority staff wherever they may be placed (e.g. Hospital based Local Authority social workers may be based on hospital premises, but are employed by the Local Authority). This is true of hands-on carers, qualified or unqualified social workers, management at all levels and those staff other than care staff such as secretaries, receptionists and porters. A circular states that all these people might need, at some time, to handle

records and have verbal contact with the clients or subjects, or the relatives of those people, in the course of their duties. It is recognised as essential that these and any others who may have personal information disclosed to them, should be aware of its sensitive nature and of their subsequent responsibility towards both subjects and information donors. They should also be made aware of the possibility of disciplinary sanctions, up to and including, dismissal for the unauthorised disclosure of information. All staff should be aware of and sign the Authority's confidentiality document. Personal information kept in a social work department should only be available to those who are directly involved in a case, including management staff, and to no others. Information is also accessible to senior managers responsible for the maintenance of good practice and standards.

16.2.2 Other Social Carers

Where an Authority has made contractual arrangements for a person's care (the example given is that of care contracted out to a voluntary organization under section 26 of the National Assistance Act 1948) or foster parents, it is recognised that those carers would require information about that person's background and history. Volunteers and informal carers might also need to be given some information about the client. It is stated that in these cases, they should undertake to be bound by Local Authority guidance on the matter.

> "*Arrangements made with others for a supply of services . . . must include adequate terms for the protection of the confidentiality of personal information.*" (Welsh Office 1989)

With regard to volunteers,

> "*any person working with a Social Services department on a voluntary basis should be subject to suitable safeguards.*" (Welsh Office 1989)

16.2.3 Other Departments of the Authority and Other Organisations

Sometimes information is needed so that the Authority may discharge its statutory functions. Some examples follow:

(a)   Finance Departments - The Authority's finance department may need some personal information to determine how much of a contribution should be made towards the cost of his own care by that individual.

(b)   Legal Staff - Information is often required when either court proceedings, or the possibility of them, arise in a case.

(c)   Child Abuse - The exchange of information is sometimes needed to prevent injury to, or abuse of a child.

(d)   The Police - Care should be taken in giving information to the police. It should be given on a "need to know" basis in the best interest of those involved.

(e)   DHSS Inspectorate - ". . . *for the purpose of their duties*" (DoH 1988).

(f)   Committee of Enquiry - may require some personal information for consideration in a case.

(g)   Cooperation with the NHS - Where it is necessary for information to be exchanged for the care of a patient/client, this is done on a reciprocal basis.

16.2.4 Management

Anonymised information is sometimes required for the administration and planning of services. Care is needed when small numbers of subjects are involved in a case, as identification can sometimes be possible by inference. At times, identifiable personal information has to be made available to the management of the Authority for ". . . *supervisory and other management purposes, the example given being that of a complaint being made against the authority or an individual officer.*" (DoH 1988)

16.2.5 Guardians ad Litem and Reporting Officers

Guardians ad litem and Reporting Officers taking part in adoption proceedings have the right under item 15 of the Adoption Agency Regulations 1983 to records held by an Adoption Agency. Where no similar right exists, the example given being of care and related proceedings, the Local Authorities are expected to allow guardians ad litem access to records, including personal information, because of that guardian ad litem's status as an officer of the court. It is also stated that access to personal information held by the Local Authority should also be given to other court officers such as probation officers, official solicitors and other such officers, to assist them in their preparation of reports for the court. The Magistrates' Courts (Adoption) Rules 1984, states that *"Any report made to the court by a guardian ad litem or a reporting officer under this rule shall remain confidential."*

16.2.6 Adoption Agencies

Although not part of the Local Authority Social Services, Adoption Agencies deal very closely with the Social Services, and social workers. These records are covered by the Access to Personal Files Act 1987. The Adoption Agency Regulations 1983 stipulate that the agency must have an adoption panel, and must include on that panel at least two social workers. Regulation 14 states that records and indexes of a case in which an adoption order was made, kept by an adoption agency in respect of both the child to be adopted and the adopter, should be kept securely for a period of at least 75 years. Regulation 15 states that all other case records should also be kept for as long as is considered appropriate.

The Regulations also stipulate that access should be given to those listed below *"as may be required"*:

(a)   those holding an enquiry under the relevant section of the Children Act 1989, for the purposes of such an enquiry

(b)   the Secretary of State

(c)   a Local Commissioner, appointed under section 23 of the Local Government Act 1974

(d)   the persons and authorities referred to in regulations 11 and 12 to the extent specified in those regulations

(e)   a Guardian ad Litem or Reporting Officer appointed for the discharge of his duties

(f)   a court having power to make an order under the various Adoption Acts or the relevant section of the Children Act 1989, for the purposes of the discharge of their duties (Adoption Agency Regulations 1983).

Part two of Regulation 15 states that an Adoption Agency may disclose such information to another Adoption Agency as it sees fit for the purposes of carrying out its functions. Regulation 16 adds that an agency may copy or transfer all or part of the record as it deems necessary in the interest of the child. Secondly, information may be disclosed to a person with the written authorization of the Secretary of State for the purposes of research. The stipulation is that a written record must be kept of any access provided, or disclosure made in respect of this regulation.

When an approved Adoption Agency ceases to act, records should be:

(a)   transferred, with the Secretary of State's permission, to another Adoption Agency

(b)   transferred to the Local Authority

(c)   in the case of an Adoption Agencies amalgamation with another Adoption Agency, transferred to the new society; in these cases the Secretary of State must be informed of this transfer.

17 The General Principles Of Confidentiality And Access Outside An Authority

The Social Services general principle of confidentiality states that personal information can be disclosed to others without their consent *"In strictly limited and exceptional cases, where the law or the public interest may override the interests of the subject"* (DoH 1988). The following are the most likely examples of occasions where personal information might be disclosed.

17.1 Courts And Tribunals

Where information is requested by a court or tribunal, information can be disclosed but this must be done strictly within the terms of the order. Consent does not need to be sought for the disclosure but the subject or donor must be notified in plenty of time for him to apply to the court or tribunal to have the order set aside, should he wish to do so.

17.2 Legislation Requiring Disclosure

Access to Personal Files Act 1987

Data Protection Act 1984

Supreme Court Rules 1981 - (Rules of the Supreme Court - Order 38)

Criminal Procedure (Attendance of Witnesses) Act 1965

Coroners Act 1988

Mental Health Review Tribunal Rules 1983

The Adoption Agency Regulations 1983

The Magistrates' Courts Act 1980

17.3 Disclosure To The Police

Some disclosures can be justified if they can help prevent, detect or prosecute a serious crime. There are however, conditions which have to be satisfied. The crime must be of a serious enough nature for its disclosure to be considered as being made in the public interest. Section 116 of the Police and Criminal Evidence Act 1984 provides some guidance. Disclosures made for this purpose should be recorded. *"It must be established that, without this disclosure the task of preventing the crime would be seriously prejudiced or delayed;"* and *". . . undertakings must be obtained that the personal information disclosed will not be used for any other purpose and will be destroyed if the person is not prosecuted, or is discharged or acquitted;*" (DoH 1988). The Social Services are also obliged to reply to a request for information from a Police Officer of the rank of superintendent or above.

Section 116 of the Police and Criminal Evidence Act 1984 defines serious crime. A "serious arrestable crime" is defined as one which might cause:

(a)   serious harm to the public order

(b)   serious harm to the security of the state

(c)   serious interference with the administration of justice

(d)   serious interference with the investigation of an offence

(e)   death

(f)   serious injury

(g)   substantial financial gain or serious financial loss.

Evidence can also at times come to the attention of staff which they feel justified in disclosing on their own initiative so as to protect another individual, the most common examples being those of child abuse and serious cases of domestic violence.

17.4 Public Health Information
It is sometimes necessary for public health information to be passed to the Proper Officer of another Local Authority. Care must be taken to ensure that this information is not subsequently used for any purpose other than that for which it was intended.

17.5 Students
Students, trainees and their college supervisors, must be made aware of the importance of confidentiality of personal information and of their duty to have regard to its sensitive and confidential nature, both during their period of training and afterwards. Both the students and their supervisors should sign the confidentiality document applicable to Local Authority staff.

17.6 Research

The Local Authority must make clients aware through policy statements, and other similar means of publicly spreading information, that their personal information can be made available on a confidential basis for the purposes of *bona fide* research. Where practical, consent should be sought for disclosure of this information. When it is not practical for permission to be sought, the Social Services department may make the decision. Written permission from the Secretary of State must be sought before researchers are allowed access to adoption information under regulation 15(2b) of the Adoption Agency Regulations 1983.

An objection by the subject or donor, made known in advance to the release of information to researchers, must at all times be respected. Each authority must establish a procedure for dealing with access by researchers, ". . . *allowing representatives from the research community to make known their views*" (DoH 1988). This procedure should also ensure that:

(a)   *"Consent to use the relevant personal information will be obtained from the Social Services department's management."* (DoH 1988)

(b)   the consent of the Local Authority is required before any approach is made to a subject or donor, as they must make the initial contact

(c)   personal information will not be disclosed to anyone outside that team of researchers and will be ". . . *adequately secured against unauthorised access.*" (DoH 1988)

(d)   published results will not enable the identification of any individual

(e)   personal information obtained for research purposes will either be destroyed within a stated period, or be archived in a non-identifiable way.

17.7 Storage And Security

The Department of Health circular, *"Personal Social Services: Confidentiality of Personal Information"* (DoH 1988), states that: *"Computer systems should be secured against unauthorised access or amendment and against loss through accidental or deliberate damage, erasure or disclosure. Failure to take reasonable care could result in an action for compensation under section 23 of the Data Protection Act 1984. Only authorised members of staff should have direct access to the case records system which should have the means for restricting the range of information needed e.g. 'passwords'. Screens of video display units should be located so that they are not open to view by unauthorised people."* In addition, *"one person in management should be made responsible for security of records in the Social Services department."* (Welsh Office 1989).

References

Adoption Agency Regulations. 1983. Statutory Instrument No. 1964. London: HMSO.

British Association of Social Workers. 1986. *A Code Of Ethics For Social Work*. Birmingham: BASW.

Department of Health. 1988. *Confidentiality Of Personal Information*. Circular LAC(88)17.

Cross, M. 27 May 1993. A Wan-dering we will go. *Health Service Journal,* pp. 35–38.

Magistrates' Courts (Adoption) Rules 1984, N0.611(L.5). London: HMSO.

Police And Criminal Evidence Act 1984. London: HMSO.

Welsh Office. 1989. *Access To Personal Files Act 1987, The Access To Personal Files (Social Services) Regulations 1989 Guidance Notes*. Circular WHC(89)5.

Draft E.C. Directive

"On the protection of individuals with regard to the processing of personal data and on the free movement of such data"

This is the second draft of the proposed Directive. The first was produced in July 1990.

The full title of the draft is:

> "Amended proposal for a *Council Directive* on the protection of individuals with regard to the processing of personal data and on the free movement of such data (presented by the Commission pursuant to Article 149(3) of the EEC Treaty)"

Its reference is COM(92) 422 final - SYN 287. It is dated 15 October 1992.

It is probable that the final Directive will only differ from this draft in a few areas, as it has been prepared in response to previous council debate and decision.

It should be noted that the proposed Directive will address the security and movement of all forms of data, and not just those relating to health and health care.

The first seven pages comprise an explanatory memorandum consequent upon the Council's adoption of its various committees' views. It is of no direct relevance here, except in one major change, which removes "... *the formal distinction between the rules applying in the public sector and the rules applying in the private sector*". Thus there will be no difference between the ways in which the data in a health service are viewed from the views taken, for example, of commercial data.

Page eight comments on changes to the title and the "Recitals". The latter are 34 statements justifying the Directive in terms of the statutory demands upon, and authority of, the European Community. Each begins with the word "whereas". If this word is removed in the reader's mind, the rest of each Recital reads in perfectly comprehensible English.

Pages 9 to 40 comment on the changes to the Articles of the Directive made as a consequence of the Council's decisions. This review is only concerned with the substance of the later draft, and will not comment on these changes.

Page 41 is the introductory page. As with all the Recitals and Articles, it is set out in two columns, with the original draft on the left and the amended draft on the right. The comments which follow refer to the latter only.

Recitals

Six of these are particularly relevant to health and health care. They read as follows:

> *"Whereas:"*

> *"(17)   data which are capable by their nature of infringing fundamental freedoms or privacy should not be processed unless the data subject gives his written consent; however, processing of these data must be permitted if it is carried out by an association the purpose of which is to help safeguard the exercise of those freedoms; on grounds of important public interest, notably in relation to the medical profession, exemptions may be granted by law or by decision of the supervisory authority laying down the limits and suitable safeguards for the processing of these types of data"*

> Comment—material likely to pose a danger to an individual must only be collected with his written consent, but some exceptions may be made, especially for doctors; the "supervisory authority" in the U.K. is the Office of the Data Protection Registrar.

*"(19)   if the processing of data is to be fair, the data subject
must be in a position to learn of the existence of a processing operation and must be given accurate and full
information where data are collected from him, and
not later than the time when the data are first disclosed
to a third party if the data subject was not informed at
the time the data were collected"*

Comment—the subject must know that data about him have
been collected, and must be told when those data
are transferred to others, and to whom.

*"(21)   the protection of the rights and freedoms of data subject
with regard to the processing of personal data requires
that appropriate technical measures be taken, both at
the time of the design of the techniques of processing
and at the time of the processing itself, particularly in
order to maintain security and thereby to prevent any
unauthorized processing"*

Comment—providing data protection as an "add-on" to a
system is inadequate and unacceptable.

*"(27)   Member States may also provide for the use of codes of
conduct drawn up by the business circles concerned
and approved by the supervisory authority, with a view
to adapting the national measures taken under this
Directive to the specific characteristics of processing in
certain sectors"*

Comment—an E.C. country may approve general rules to
enable different sectors (e.g. the NHS) to adopt
the Directive's requirements uniformly.

*"(28)   Member States must encourage the business circles
concerned to draw up Community codes of conduct so
as to facilitate the application of this Directive; the
Commission will support such initiatives and will take
them into account when it considers the appropriate-*

ness of additional specific measures in respect of certain sectors"

Comment—an E.C. country must encourage its businesses and sectors to undertake the work specified in Recital 27.

"(30)   at Community level, a Working Party on the Protection of Individuals with regard to the Processing of Personal Data must be set up and be completely independent in the performance of its functions; . . . it must advise the Commission and, in particular, contribute to the uniform application of the national rules adopted pursuant to this Directive"

Comment—a watchdog Working Party is to be set up to ensure Member State compliance.

Articles

Chapter I General Provisions
Article 2 Definitions

"(a)   "personal data" means any information relating to an identified or identifiable natural person ("data subject"); an identifiable person is one who can be identified, directly or indirectly, in particular by reference to an identification number or to one or more factors specific to his physical, physiological, mental, economic, cultural or social identity;

data presented in statistical form, which is of such a type that the persons concerned can no longer be reasonably identified are not considered as personal data"

Comment—subject identifiability, by any means, is the test by which the existence of personal data must be determined.

"(b)   *"processing of personal data" ("processing") means any*
        operation or set of operations which is performed upon
        personal data, whether or not by automatic means . . ."

Comment—this directive does not restrict itself to electroni-
        cally held data (Article 3 indicates this more fully,
        and states the exceptions to wit - activities
        outside the scope of Community law, and purely
        private and personal activities).

"(c)   *"personal data file" ("file") means any structured set of*
        personal data, whether centralized or geographically
        dispersed, which is accessible according to specific
        criteria and whose object or effect is to facilitate the use
        or alignment of data relating to the data subject or
        subjects"

Comment—three features count in the definition of a "file" -
        structure, accessibility, and the intent to use it or
        to gain in understanding of its data content.

"(d)   *"controller" means any natural or legal person, public*
        authority, agency or other body who processes personal
        data or causes it to be processed and who decides what
        is the purpose and objective of the processing, which
        personal data are to be processed, which operations are
        to be performed upon them and which third parties are
        to have access to them;

Comment—in the U.K. the controller equates to the Data Pro-
        tection Officer of an organisation.

"(g)   *"the data subject's consent" means any express indica-*
        tion of his wishes by which the data subject signifies
        his agreement to personal data relating to him being
        processed, on condition he has available information
        about the purposes of the processing, the data or
        categories of data concerned, the recipient of the
        personal data, and the name and address of the
        controller and of his representative if any;

The data subject's consent must be freely given and specific, and may be withdrawn by the data subject at any time, but without retrospective effect"

Comment—consent need not in principle be written (but see Article 8); it must be informed, and it can be withdrawn.

Chapter 11 General Rules On the Lawfulness Of The Processing Of Personal Data

Section I Principles Relating To Data Quality
Article 6

"1   *Member States shall provide that personal data must be:*

(a)   *processed fairly and lawfully;*

(b)   *collected for specified, explicit and legitimate purposes and used in a way compatible with those purposes;*

(c)   *adequate, relevant and not excessive in relation to the purposes for which they are processed;*

(d)   *accurate and, where necessary, kept up to date; every step must be taken to ensure that data which are inaccurate or incomplete having regard to the purposes for which they were collected are erased or rectified;*

(e)   *kept in a form which permits identification of data subjects for no longer than is necessary for the purposes in view; Member States may lay down appropriate safeguards for personal data stored for historical, statistical or scientific use.*

Comment—this article states many of the requirements of "fair obtaining" already enshrined in the Data Protection Act 1984 (q.v.); the last clause, permitting the safeguarding of data for research uses, is of particular relevance to the NHS research community.

Section II Principles Relating To The Grounds For Processing Data

Article 7

> *"Member States shall provide that personal data may be processed only if:*
>
> *(a)   the data subject has consented;*
>
> *(b)   processing is necessary for the performance of a contract with the data subject, or in order to take steps at the request of the data subject preliminary to entering into a contract;*
>
> *(c)   processing is necessary in order to comply with an obligation imposed by national law or by Community law;*
>
> *(d)   processing is necessary in order to protect the vital interests of the data subject;*
>
> *(e)   processing is necessary for the performance of a task in the public interest or carried out in the exercise of public authority vested in the controller or in a third party to whom the data are disclosed; or*
>
> *(f)   processing is necessary in pursuit of the general interest or of the legitimate interests of the controller or of a third party to whom the data are disclosed, except where such interests are overridden by the interests of the data subject."*

Comment—the range of principles is large, and wholly governed by the crucial word "or" (clause [e]) which allows any one of them to be cited; note that clauses [b] to [f] may all operate even in the absence of consent by the data subject (because of the "or").

Section III Special Categories Of Processing

Article 8   The processing of special categories of data

> *"1   Member States shall prohibit the processing of data revealing racial or ethnic origin, political opinions,*

religious beliefs, philosophical or ethical persuasion or trade-union membership, and of data concerning health and sexual life"

Comment—this clause is inserted to offset the principles stated in Article 7, requiring special consideration of the data subject's wishes in special cases; the following clauses modify its uncompromising nature.

"2   *Member States shall provide that data referred to in paragraph 1 may be processed where:*

(a)   *the data subject has given his written consent to the processing of that data, except where the laws of the Member State provide that the prohibition referred to in paragraph 1 may not be waived by the data subject giving his consent;*

(b)   *processing is carried out by a foundation or non-profit-making association of a political, philosophical, religious or trade-union character in the course of its legitimate activities and on condition that the processing relates solely to members of the foundation or association and to persons who have regular contact with it in connection with its purposes and that the data are not disclosed to third parties without the data subject's consent; or*

(c)   *the processing is performed in circumstances where there is manifestly no infringement of privacy or fundamental freedoms.*

Comment—clause 2[a] requires written consent before health data may be collected; the U.K. has no legislation specifically prohibiting collection of the data items listed in clause 1; clause 2[c] appears to require testing in the courts for it to be clarified under English common law.

"3   Member States may, on grounds of important public interest, lay down exemptions from paragraph 1 by national legislative provision or by decision of the supervisory authority, stating the types of data which may be processed, the persons to whom such data may be disclosed and the persons who may be controllers, and specifying suitable safeguards."

Comment—the Office of the Data Protection Registrar is, by this clause, empowered to exempt specific data types from the general prohibition; whether it feels it is empowered to do so under existing U.K. legislation will become clear under test.

"5   Member States shall determine the conditions under which a national identification number or other identifier of general application may be used.

Comment—the use of the new NHS number falls within the provisions of this clause.

Section IV Information To Be Given To The Data Subject

Article 10 The existence of a processing operation

"1   Member States shall ensure that any person is entitled, on request, to know of the existence of a processing operation. . . ." (there follows details of what should be disclosed, as follows in article 11).

Comment—this provision is already contained within the Data Protection Act 1984.

Article 11 Collection of data from the data subject

"1   Member States shall provide that the controller must ensure that a data subject from whom data are collected be informed at least of the following:

(a)   the purposes of the processing for which the data are intended;

(b)   the obligatory or voluntary nature of any reply to the questions to which answers are sought;

(c)   *the consequences for him if he fails to reply;*

(d)   *the recipients or categories of recipients of the data;*

(e)   *the existence of a right of access to and rectification of the data relating to him; and*

(f)   *the name and address of the controller and of his representative, if any."*

Comment—within the field of health and health care, and under the Data Protection Act 1984, the collection of data from the subject is in general voluntary, and the consequences of failure to reply, except where the public interest is at stake (as in an outbreak of communicable disease, for example) are those of a poorer quality of individual care; the right of access to the data may only be withheld in special circumstances under the Act.

Section V The Data Subject's Right Of Access To Data

Article 13 Right of Access

"1   (second para) *Member States may provide that the right of access to medical data may be exercised only through a medical practitioner"*

Comment—this is the likeliest route of access, but the enabling nature of this clause should be noted; some health care practitioners other than doctors practice in their own right, collect health (if not always medical) data unrelated to those collected by doctors, and thus are likely to be the route through which such data are accessed by the data subject.

Article 14 Exemptions to the right of access

"1   *Unless obliged to do so by a provision of Community law, Member States may restrict the exercise of the rights provided for in Article 10(1) and in point 1 of*

Article 13 where such restriction is necessary to safe-guard:

(a)   *national security;*

(b)   *defence;*

(c)   *criminal proceedings;*

(d)   *public safety;*

(e)   *a duly established paramount economic and financial interest of a Member State or of the Community;*

(f)   *a monitoring or inspection function performed by a public authority or an activity undertaken to assist the performance of such a function;*

(g)   *an equivalent right of another person and the rights and freedoms of others."*

Comment—these are standard exception clauses in many documents of this kind, where the exemption cited may be challenged in the courts; the commentary to the articles states, in relation to clause 1[e]. *"The phrase 'substantial economic and financial interests of the Member State or of the European Communities' refers to all economic policy measures and measures to finance the policies of a Member State or the Community, such as exchange controls, foreign trade controls, and tax collection. But only a substantial interest of this kind would justify a restriction of the right of access"* - this is unlikely to be the case in health care, and in relation to disclosure to an individual data subject.

Section VII Security Of Processing

This section deals with what is now referred to in the U.K. as "Physical Security", and requires a certain minimum standard for protecting data from unauthorised access.

Chapter III Judicial Remedies, Liability And Penalties

Article 22 Judicial Remedies

> *"Member States shall provide for the right of every person to a judicial remedy for any breach of the rights guaranteed by this Directive."*

> Comment—this requires only a small alteration to U K law as it stands.

The Article and clauses reviewed above are those most relevant to health and health care in the United Kingdom. Many of the provisions proposed for the Directive already exist in the Data Protection Act 1984. Some elements of the Directive, however, will create a requirement for changes to the Act, in particular those pertaining to the need to obtain written consent to the collection of *"data concerning health or sexual life"*. Such a requirement may have serious consequences for the practice of epidemiology, and other potentially multi-centred research projects. Proof of *"impor-tant public interest"* may have to be provided to allow some of these types of work to proceed.

The proposal suggests that Member States be allowed three years from the passage of the Directive for its implementation.

Recent verbal commentary (as of July 1994) suggests that the modifications to Article 8 have been substantially strengthened to enable health data, in particular, to be collected more easily. Additionally, a clause permitting the retention of health data, for research purposes, for longer than specifically needed for the care of the subject, is to be inserted.

Glossary

Access

Authorisation which permits an individual to use a resource (including to see clinical material) which has been deemed to be subject to Access Control.

Access Control

Prevention of unauthorised use of a resource, including the prevention of use of a resource in an unauthorised manner. (ISO 7498-2)

Availability

Property of being accessible and usable upon demand by an authorised entity. (ISO 7498-2)

Prevention of the unauthorised withholding of information or resources. (European ITSEC)

Assurance

Confidence that may be held in the security provided by a Target of Evaluation. (European ITSEC)

Confidentiality

Set of rules governing restricted material by which individuals are given or refused access authority.

Clinician

Qualified professional attendant upon an individual patient in his or her professional capacity (i.e. including medical, nursing, paramedical and other relevant disciplines).

Integrity

Prevention of unauthorised modification of information. (European ITSEC)

Patient

Individual receiving health care services, or for whom such services are available.

Physical Security

Measures used to provide physical protection of resources against deliberate and accidental threats. (ISO 74980-2)

Privacy

Right of individuals to control or influence what information related to them may be collected and stored and by whom that information may be disclosed. (ISO 7498-2)

Security

Combination of confidentiality, integrity and availability (q.v.). (European ITSEC)

Target of Evaluation

System under test for the quality of its security (q.v.).

Threat

Action or event that might prejudice security. (European ITSEC)

Vulnerability

Security weakness in a Target of Evaluation due to failures in analysis, design, implementation or operation. (European ITSEC)

Bibliography

General

Allaërt, F. A. & Dusserre, L. 1992. "Transborder Flows Of Personal Medical Data In Europe: Legal And Ethical Approach". *MEDINFO 92*. K. C. Lun *et al.* (Editors). North-Holland: Elsevier Science Publishers B.V.

Barber, B. & Davey, J. 1991. *The Use Of The CCTA Risk Analysis And Management Methodology [CRAMM] In Health Information Systems*.

Barber, B., Vincent, R. & Scholes, M. 1991. *Worst Case Scenarios: The Legal & Ethical Imperative*. Birmingham: NHS Information Management Centre.

Barber, B. 1991. *The European Community's Safety First Principles For Health Information Systems*. Birmingham: NHS Information Management Centre.

Barber, B. 1991. *Towards An Information Technology Security Policy For The NHS*. Birmingham: NHS Information Management Centre.

Bengtsson, S. & Solheim, B. G. 1992. Enforcement Of Data Protection, Privacy And Security In Medical Informatics. *MEDINFO 92*. K. C. Lun *et al.* (Editors). North-Holland: Elsevier Science Publishers B.V.

Brannigan, V. M. 1992. Protecting the Privacy of Patient Information in Clinical Networks: Regulatory Effectiveness Analysis. *Annals New York Academy of Sciences*: 190–201.

British Association Of Social Workers. 1986. *A Code Of Ethics For Social Work*. BASW.

British Medical Association. 1991. *Guidelines For Doctors On The Access To Health Records Act 1990*. BMA.

British Medical Association. 1992. *Rights And Responsibilities Of Doctors*. London: BMJ Publishing Group.

British Medical Association. 1993. *Confidentiality & People Under 16*. London: BMA.

British Paediatric Association, Ethics Advisory Committee. August 1992. *Guidelines For The Ethical Conduct Of Medical Research Involving Children*. London: BPA.

British Psychological Society (Division Of Clinical Psychology). 1990. *Guidelines For The Professional Practice Of Clinical Psychology*. Leicester: BPS.

British Psychological Society. 1993. *Code of Conduct, Ethical Principles & Guidelines*. Leicester: BPS.

Burnard, P. & Chapman, C. M. 1988. *Professional And Ethical Issues In Nursing. The Code Of Professional Conduct*. Chichester: Wiley.

Commission Of The European Communities. 15 October 1992. Amended Proposal For A Council Directive On The Protection Of Individuals With Regard To The Processing Of Personal Data And On The Free Movement Of Such Data. Brussels: COM (92) 422 final - SYN 287.

Commission Of The European Communities DG XIII/FAIM, 1991. Data Protection And Confidentiality In Health Informatics. Handling Health Data In Europe In The Future. IOS Press.

Committee on Improving the Patient Record Division of Health Care Services. 1991. *The Computer-Based Patient Record*. Dick, R. S. & Steen, E. B. (Editors). Washington DC: National Academy Press.

Computers & Security. December 1992. *Elsevier Advanced Technology*, Vol. 11, No. 8.

Conference of Medical Royal Colleges and their Faculties in the United Kingdom. Interim Guidelines on Confidentiality and Medical Audit. 14 December 1991. *British Medical Journal*, Vol. 303, p. 1525.

Council of Europe. 1981. Explanatory Report On The Convention For The Protection Of Individuals With Regard To Automatic Processing Of Personal Data. Strasbourg: Council of Europe, IST/35/-6/51.

Council of Europe. 1981. Regulations For Automated Medical Data Banks. Strasbourg: Council of Europe, IST/35/-6/52.

Council for Professions Supplementary to Medicine. August & October 1993. *Infamous Conduct Statements*. London: CPSM.

Cross, M. 15 April 1993. Big Brother. *Health Service Journal*, pp. 20–22.

Cross, M. 8 July 1993. Protect And Survive. *Health Service Journal*, p. 8.

Data Protection Registrar. 1988. Fourth Report of The Data Protection Registrar. London: HMSO.

Data Protection Registrar. March 1992. Guidelines To The Data Protection Act 1984, Data Protection, Nos 1–8. The Office of the Data Protection Registrar.

Data Protection Registrar. 27 October 1993. Account 1991–92. London: HMSO.

Data Protection Registrar. February 1993. "NHS Contract Minimum Data Sets" The Office of the Data Protection Registrar.

Data Protection Registrar. 1993. Ninth Report Of The Data Protection Registrar. London: HMSO.

Department of Health. September 1988. Personal Social Services: Confidentiality Of Personal Information. DoH.

Department of Health. 1990. Medical Audit: Guidance For Hospital Clinicians On The Use Of Computers. DoH.

Department of Health. January 1991. Medical Audit: In The Hospital And Community Health Services, Assuring The Quality Of Medical Care: Implementation Of Medical & Dental Audit In The Hospital And Community Health Services. DoH.

Department of Health and Social Security. September 1982. Health Services Management: Supply Of Information About Hospital Patients In The Context Of Civil Legal Proceedings. DHSS.

Department of Health and Social Security. 3 September 1985. Data Protection Act: Subject Access To Personal Health Information. DHSS.

Department of Health and Social Security. 2 March 1988. Protection Of Children: Disclosure Of Criminal Background Of Those With Access To Children. DHSS.

Everette, A. *et al.* 1986. Medical Image Management: Practical, Legal And Ethical Considerations. *Computers In Biology And Medicine*, Volume 16, pp. 247–257.

Galloway, Mandy. 28 March 1991. Why Patients May Put Privacy Issue On Trial. *Doctor*, p. 34.

Gardner, Elizabeth. 3 November 1989. Computer Dilemma: Clinical Access vs Confidentiality. *Modern Health Care*, pp. 32–42.

General Medical Council. December 1993. *Professional Conduct And Discipline: Fitness To Practise*. London: GMC.

Godber, P. May 1981. Confidentiality Of Case Records. *The Health Visitor*, Vol. 54, p. 193.

Griew, A. R., Darley, B. S. & McLoughlin, K. S. 1994. The Electronic Transfer Of Clinical Records: Suggested Rules To Control Access And Confidentiality. In *Current Perspectives in Healthcare Computing 1994*. Richards, B. (Editor). Weybridge: BJHC.

Gritzalis, D. & Katsikas, S. 1992. Data Confidentiality And User Access Rights In Medical Information Systems. *MEDINFO 92*. K. C. Lun *et al.* (Editors). North-Holland: Elsevier Science Publishers B.V.

Harding, N. G. L. (ed). 1986. *Data Protection In Medicine*. Oxford: University Computing Service.

Hawker, Andrew. 24 September 1992. Deus Ex Machina. *Health Service Journal*, pp. 28–29.

Health & Safety Commission. 1985. Discussion Document: Access To Health And Safety Information By Members Of The Public. Health & Safety Commission.

Health & Safety Commission. 1987. Health And Safety Commission Policy Statement On Access To Health And Safety Information By Members Of The Public. Health & Safety Commission.

Hoyte, P. August 1993. *Can I See The Records?* Medical Defence Union.

Institute Of Medicine. 1991. *The Computer-Based Patient Record - An Essential Technology For Health Care.* National Academy Press.

International Medical Informatics Association, Working Group 4. November 1993. Caring for Health Information Safety, Security and Secrecy. Preprints of conference papers, IMIA.

Jackson, A. D. M. March 1986. Confidentiality And Paediatric Practice. *Archives Of Disease In Childhood*, Vol. 61, No. 3, pp. 303–304.

Jones, Jeffrey R. December 1991. Patients' Access To Their Psychiatric Notes: A Review. *Psychiatric Bulletin*, Vol. 15, No. 12, pp. 753–754.

Körner, E. October 1984. The Protection and Maintenance of Confidentiality of Patient and Employee Data. A Report From the Confidentiality Working Group. Steering Group on Health Services Information. HMSO, London.

Koska, Mary T. 5 January 1992. Outcomes Research: Hospitals Face Confidentiality Concerns. *Hospitals*, pp. 32–34..

Martin, D. 31 March 1993. Access Control to Medical Records Working Group 5 - Proposals for Prototypes and Test Sites. Brussels: AIM/CEN Workshop on HCR.

Medical Defence Union. January 1992. *Confidentiality.* London: MDU.

Medical Defence Union. April 1992. *Medical Records.* London: MDU.

Medical Protection Society. 1991. *Consent And Confidentiality.* London: MPS.

Medical Protection Society. 1991. *Statutory Notifications To Public Authorities, Reporting Deaths To Coroners, The Mental Health Act 1983.* London: MPS.

Medical Protection Society. 1992. *Disclosure Of Medical Records.* London: MPS.

Medical Records Institute. January 1993. Computerization And Confidentiality. *Towards An Electronic Patient Record - Updates On Standards And Developments*, Vol. 1, No. 6. PO Box 289, Newton, MA 02160: Medical Records Institute.

Medical Research Council. 1985. *Responsibility In The Use Of Personal Information For Research - Principles And Guide To Practice*. MRC.

Medical Research Council. November 1992. *Responsibility In Investigations On Human Participants And Material And On Personal Information*. MRC.

Millar, Barbara. 30 May 1991. Sharing The Caring. *The Health Service Journal*, pp. 33–34.

Naish, Jane & Barr, Melanie. 1991. Rights Of Access. *Health Visitor Journal*, Vol. 64, No. 9, pp. 300–301.

National Council for Civil Liberties. October 1987. Your Right To See Your File. *Civil Liberty*.

NHS Information Management Group. 1990. Working For Patients. Framework For Information Systems: Overview Working Paper 11. London: HMSO.

NHS Management Executive. 1991. Access To Health Records Act 1990, A Guide For The NHS. NHSME.

NHS Management Executive. 1992. Information Systems Security: Top Level Policy For The NHS. NHSME.

NHS Management Executive. 1992. Basic Information Systems Security. NHSME.

NHS Management Executive. December 1992. Information System Security And You. NHSME.

NHS Management Executive. October 1993. Making An Informed Choice. NHSME.

NHS Wales. 1991/1992. The Medical Record Commandments. Medical Records Forum.

Panting, Gerard. September 1991. The Access To Health Records Act 1990. *Practise Nurse*, pp. 206–209.

Payne, R. H. 1992. *Professional Discipline In Nursing, Midwifery And Health Visiting.* 2nd ed. Oxford: Blackwell Scientific Publications.

Rigby, M., McBride, A. & Shiels, C. *Computers In Medical Audit.* 2nd ed. London: Royal Society of Medicine.

Robertson, C. 1991. *Health Visiting In Practice.* 2nd ed. Edinburgh: Churchill Livingstone.

Robinson, David M. 1992. A Legal Examination Of Format, Signature And Confidentiality Aspects Of Computerized Health Information. *MEDINFO 92.* K. C. Lun *et al.* (Editors). North Holland: Elsevier Science Publishers B.V.

Robinson, K. & Vaughan, B. 1992. *Knowledge For Nursing Practise.* Oxford: Butterworth Heinemann.

Royal College Of Nursing. November 1992. *Response To Guidance On NHS Staff Freedom Of Speech.* London: RCN.

Royal College Of Nursing. March 1993. Issues In Nursing And Health - Fact Sheets 1–12, 14–19. London: RCN.

Royal College Of Obstetrians And Gynaecologists. November 1982. *Statement On Confidentiality.* London: RCOG.

Scally, Gabriel. 6 November 1993. Confidentiality, contraception, and young people. *British Medical Journal,* Vol. 307, pp. 1157–1158.

Schuchman, H., Foster, L. & Nye, S. 1982. S. *Confidentiality of Health Records.* Gardner Press.

Select Committee On The European Communities. 30 March 1993. Protection Of Personal Data. London: HMSO.

Tew, Jo & Deadman, Nadia. 25 March 1993. Parent Power. *Health Service Journal,* p. 31.

The Computer Law and Security Report. May–June 1993. *Elsevier Advanced Technology,* Vol. 9, Issue 3.

Tonks, A. 13 November 1993. Information Management And Patient Privacy In The NHS. *British Medical Journal,* Vol. 307, pp. 1227–1228.

Treacher, A., Barber, B. & Osborne, D. 1992. *Training For Health Information Security: An Approach To Cultural Change*. Birmingham: NHS Information Management Centre.

United Kingdom Central Council for Nursing, Midwifery and Health Visiting. March 1989. *Exercising Accountability*. London: UKCC.

United Kingdom Central Council for Nursing, Midwifery and Health Visiting. June 1992. *Code Of Professional Conduct*. London: UKCC.

United Kingdom Central Council for Nursing, Midwifery and Health Visiting. 1987. *Confidentiality: An Elaboration of Clause 9 of the Second Edition of the UKCC's Code of Professional Conduct for the Nurse, Midwife and Health Visitor*. London: UKCC.

Vaughan, B. & Pillmore, M. (Editors). 1989. *Managing Nursing Work*. London: Scutari Press.

Wadeley, A. 1991. *Ethics In Psychological Research And Practice*. British Psychological Society Books.

Watson, D 1985. *A Code Of Ethics For Social Work, The Second Step*. London: Routledge & Kegan Paul.

Welsh Office. August 1976. Health Services Management Medical Evidence For Social Security Purposes. Cardiff: Welsh Office.

Welsh Office. May 1976. Health Services Management Protection Of Commercially Valuable Information. Cardiff: Welsh Office.

Welsh Office. June 1977. Health Services Development: The Role Of Psychologists In The Health Service Summary. Cardiff: Welsh Office.

Welsh Office. July 1980. Health Services Management Confidentiality Of Medical Records. Cardiff: Welsh Office.

Welsh Office. February 1982. Health Services Development: Professional Advisory Machinery: Professions Other Than Medicine. Cardiff: Welsh Office.

Welsh Office. September 1982. Health Services Management: Supply Of Information About Hospital Patients In The Context Of Civil Legal Proceedings. Cardiff: Welsh Office.

Welsh Office. January 1983. Health Services Management: Security. Cardiff: Welsh Office.

Welsh Office. September 1983. Health Services Development: Direction NHS Act 1977. Cardiff: Welsh Office.

Welsh Office. March 1985. Health Services Management: The Public Health (Infectious Diseases) Regulations 1985. Cardiff: Welsh Office.

Welsh Office. June 1985. Development Of An Information, Computing And Communications Strategy In The NHS In Wales. Cardiff: Welsh Office.

Welsh Office. September 1985. Data Protection Act: Subject Access To Personal Health Information. Cardiff: Welsh Office.

Welsh Office. 26 September 1987. Data Protection Act 1984: Modified Access To Personal Health Information. Cardiff: Welsh Office.

Welsh Office. 31 October 1986. OPREN - Disclosure Of Medical Records. Cardiff: Welsh Office.

Welsh Office. 17 December 1987. Health Service Management Data Protection Act 1984: Modified Access To Personal Health Information. Cardiff: Welsh Office.

Welsh Office. 16 March 1989. Community Health Councils (Access To Information) Act 1988. Cardiff: Welsh Office.

Welsh Office. 17 November 1989. Health Services Management Data Protection Act 1984: Modified Access To Personal Health Information. Cardiff: Welsh Office.

Welsh Office. 17 August 1990. NHS Review - "Working For Patients" Medical Audit In The Family Practitioner Services. Cardiff: Welsh Office.

Welsh Office. 18 Septemer 1990. Patient Consent To Examination Or Treatment. Cardiff: Welsh Office.

Welsh Office. 4 January 1991. Referrals By General Medical Practitioners: Information Requirements For 1991/92. Cardiff: Welsh Office.

Welsh Office. April 1991. Medical Students In Hospitals. Cardiff: Welsh Office.

Welsh Office. 22 April 1991. Confidentiality Of Personal Health Data. Cardiff: Welsh Office.

Welsh Office. 24 July 1991. Access To Personal Files (Social Services) (Amendment) Regulations 1991. Cardiff: Welsh Office.

Welsh Office. 4 September 1991. The Access To Health Records Act 1990 (with NHSME guide). Cardiff: Welsh Office.

Welsh Office. 23 Septemer 1991. Local Research Ethics Committees. Cardiff: Welsh Office.

Westcott. R. & Jones. R. V. H. 1988. *Information Handling In General Practice, Challenges For The Future.* London: Croom Helm.

Wright, Stephen. 5 December 1990. Patients' Access To Nursing Records. *Nursing Standard*, Vol. 5, No. 11, pp. 22–24.

Ying Hui Tan. 8 June 1993. No Right Of Access To Health Records. Law Report. *Independent Newspaper.*

Legislation

Abortion Act 1967.

Access To Health Records Act 1990.

Access To Health Reports Act 1988.

Access To Personal Files Act 1987.

Adoption Act 1976.

AIDS (Control) Act 1987.

Anatomy Act 1984.

Births and Deaths Registration Act 1953.

Census Act 1920 (as amended).

Children Act 1989.

Community Health Councils (Access To Information) Act 1988.

Computer Misuse Act 1990.

Copyright, Designs And Patents Act 1988.

Data Protection Act 1984.

Environment And Safety Information Act 1988.

Health Service Joint Consultative Committees (Access To Information) Act 1986.

Health Services Act 1976.

Health Services & Public Health Act 1968.

Housing Act 1985.

Human Fertilisation and Embryology (Disclosure of Information) Act 1992.

Human Organ Transplant Act 1989.

Human Tissue Act 1961.

Local Government Act 1974.

Medical Act 1983.

Mental Health Act 1983.

Misuse Of Drugs Act 1971.

National Assistance Act 1948 (as amended).

NHS Act 1977.

NHS Community Care Act 1990.

Police And Criminal Evidence Act 1984.

Population (Statistics) Act 1938.

Prevention Of Terrorism (Temporary Provisions) Act 1976.

Professions Supplementary To Medicine Act 1960.

Public Bodies (Admission To Meetings) Act 1960.

Public Health Act 1936, 1961.

Public Health (Control of Disease) Act 1984.

Public Records Act 1958.

Road Traffic Act 1972.

Still-Birth (Definition) Act 1992.

Supreme Court Act 1981 plus The Rules Of The Supreme Court 1965.

Venereal Disease Act 1917.

Statutory Instruments

Children And Young Persons (The Adoption Agencies Regulations) 1983.

Children And Young Persons (The Adoption Rules) 1984.

Education, England And Wales (The Education (Special Educational Needs) Regulations) 1983.

Health And Safety (Emissions Into The Atmosphere) Regulations 1983.

Magistrates' Courts (The Magistrates' Courts (Adoption) Rules) 1984.

Mental Health (Hospital, Guardianship And Consent To Treatment) Regulations 1983.

Public Health (Infectious Diseases) Regulations 1985.

Residential Care Homes Regulations 1984 (Social Welfare Services).

Subject Access Modification (Health) Order 1987

Case Law

Attorney General v *Guardian Newspapers Ltd* (No2) [1988] 3 All ER 545

D v *NSPCC* [1977] 1 All ER 589

Gillick v *Norfolk and Wisbech Area Health Authority* [1985] 3 WLR 830, 3 All ER 402

Hunter v *Mann* [1974] 2 All ER 414

Rice v *Connolly* [1966] 2 All ER 649

W v *Egdell* [1990] 1 All ER 835

X v *Y* [1988] 2 All ER 648

R v *Mid-Glamorgan Family Health Services Authority* [1993] 137 SJ 153

Printed in the United Kingdom for HMSO
Dd 297848 C10 10/94 9091